MW01614447

the IBD REMISSION Diet

Achieving long-term health with an elemental diet & natural supplementation plan

Jini Patel Thompson

CARAMAL PUBLISHING

Also by Jini Patel Thompson

LISTEN TO YOUR GUT: Natural Healing & Dealing with Inflammatory Bowel Disease & Irritable Bowel Syndrome

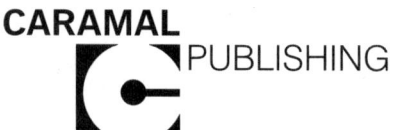

CARAMAL PUBLISHING

the IBD REMISSION Diet

Achieving long-term health with an elemental diet & natural supplementation plan

Crohn's • Ulcerative Colitis • Diverticulitis
• Irritable Bowel Syndrome

Jini Patel Thompson

Caramal Publishing Inc.
P.O. Box 29022,
Vancouver, B.C.,
V6J 5C2, Canada

National Library of Canada Cataloguing in Publication Data
Thompson, Jini Patel, 1968-
The IBD remission diet : achieving long-term health with an elemental diet & natural supplementation plan : Crohn's, ulcerative colitis, diverticulitis, irritable bowel syndrome / Jini Patel Thompson.

Includes bibliographical references and index.
ISBN 0-9685421-2-3

1. Inflammatory bowel diseases--Diet therapy. 2. Inflammatory bowel diseases--Alternative treatment. 3. Colon (Anatomy)--Diseases--Diet therapy. 4. Colon (Anatomy)--Diseases--Alternative treatment.
5. Elemental diet. I. Title.
RC862.I53T45 2003   616.3'4   C2002-911084-X

Printed in Canada
First Edition

Cover Design by Mariana Prins
Book Design by Mariana Prins
Cover Photo by Jud Lewis-Mahon

DISCLAIMER

This book is designed to provide information in regard to the subject matter covered. It is sold with the understanding that the publisher and author are not engaged in rendering medical, naturopathic, homeopathic or other professional services. If medical or other expert assistance is required, the services of a competent professional should be sought. Every effort has been made to make this book as complete and accurate as possible. However, there may be mistakes both typographical and in content. Therefore this book should be used only as a general guide and not as the ultimate source of information on intestinal health. Furthermore, this book contains information on IBD/IBS only up to the printing date. The purpose of this book is to educate and entertain. The author and Caramal Publishing shall have neither liability nor responsibility to any person or entity with respect to any loss or damage caused, or alleged to be caused, directly or indirectly by the information contained in this book. If you do not wish to be bound by this disclaimer, you may return this book to the publisher within 30 days of purchase for a full refund.

*To my wonderful mother, Anita, and my
husband, Ian, who supported me through the research,
encouraged me, made the broths, and
whipped up shakes tirelessly!
My success in health is yours as well as mine.*

ACKNOWLEDGEMENTS

With many thanks to Dr. Frank H. Anderson MD (GI) and Jerry Cyr RN, at Vancouver General Hospital, who first introduced me to the concept of an elemental diet. Thanks also to the tireless editors of this book: Mary & Tony Macer, Dr. Sharad Patel, Anita Patel, and Ian Thompson - you've all made this a better book than it was originally. Also many thanks to Emily Donaldson for excellent feedback and valuable, clarifying questions on the manuscript.

TABLE OF CONTENTS

1

THE STORY
& THE VISION

*Do not go where the path may lead,
go instead where there is no path and leave a trail.*

Ralph Waldo Emerson

THE IBD REMISSION DIET is a very specific natural diet and supplementation plan devised to induce disease remission; by completely healing the gastrointestinal tract, starving off all the bacteria in your intestine and replacing them with good bacteria, and restoring health and balance from the cellular level on up throughout the immune system. Although it is specifically formulated to address inflammatory bowel conditions like Crohn's, Ulcerative Colitis and Diverticulitis, you will probably find other health problems will also be resolved as the program facilitates extensive whole body healing.

My previous book, *LISTEN TO YOUR GUT: Natural Healing & Dealing With Inflammatory Bowel Disease & Irritable Bowel Syndrome*, (available at www.caramal.com) contains a section on using an elemental diet to induce disease remission or test for food allergies. However, feedback from readers told me they wanted more. Following an elemental diet is a difficult undertaking requiring a lot of self-discipline and they wanted more information on the basis and reasoning behind the diet and also more detailed instructions on implementation. This book provides both and I have also extended the elemental diet to include my whole-body-healing supplementation plan. If you're going to undertake something as difficult and restrictive as an elemental diet, then you might as well fully commit to it and use this period to facilitate a complete overhaul and root-level healing of your body and immune system. And who knows, many of you may even experience the C-word (cure!) as a result.

Recent clinical trials involving children with active Crohn's disease in England and Italy have demonstrated that "elemental diet therapy is as effective as steroids in inducing remission, whilst avoiding steroid side effects" (Dr. Bhupinder Sandhu). In the English study, 44 children with Crohn's were put on an elemental diet and 40 of them (90%) achieved clinical remission in an average of 6 weeks (individual times on the elemental diet ranged from 2 - 12 weeks). In the Italian study, 37 children were assigned to an elemental diet and 10 children were assigned methylprednisone (steroids). Thirty-two (86%) of the children on the elemental diet achieved clinical remission in an average of 2.5 weeks and 9 of the children on steroids achieved clinical remission in an average of 3.7 weeks. However, 7 of the children on the elemental diet showed complete healing of the mucosal lining of the intestine, while none of the children on steroids showed healing of the mucosal lining. As Dr. Robert Canani summarized: "In children with active Crohn's disease, exclusive nutritional therapy shows a more rapid effect than steroids in inducing clinical remission and is markedly more effective than steroids in producing healing of mucosal inflammation." (*DDW Annual Meeting: Abstracts 103976, 107178. May 19 & 21, 2002*)

I have gone on an elemental diet twice in my life. The first time was due to intestinal haemorrhaging that left me at 99 lbs (I'm 5'7") and required a transfusion of 6 pints of blood. I had two objectives; stop the bleeding and gain weight. Continuing to eat regular food simply re-opened the wounds and started the bleeding again. Therefore, my nutrition needed to come from a completely pre-digested (elemental) liquid source, which my gastroenterologist told me resulted in disease remission as often as Prednisone (steroids). I sampled each of the elemental (pre-digested) products provided by the hospital, but found the taste and ingredient list unacceptable. All of the products contained artificial flavors and sweeteners, large amounts of sugar (in relation to maltodextrin) and high levels of low quality oils - which resulted in painful intestinal spasming. Rather than drinking these, or, undergoing a surgical procedure to have a tube inserted in my stomach and the commercial elemental products pumped in, I set out to find a natural, healthy alternative.

After an extensive search of health stores and the Internet, I devised my own elemental formula by mixing together 6 different products. I did this 8-9 times a day to give my body the nutrients it needed in elemental (pre-digested for maximum absorption) form. Because all the food I ate (or more accurately, drank) was pre-digested, the elemental diet also gave my bowel a complete rest, which allowed my wounds time and space to heal. In addition, I added numerous supplements to each shake to further facilitate my healing and recovery. Using this formula, I gained 36 pounds of solid weight (not fat) in six weeks and my albumin (blood protein) levels were restored to normal. I went from being so weak I could barely move around my apartment, to cycling and lifting weights at the gym at a solid weight of 135 lbs. One month later I got pregnant, had an excellent pregnancy and gave birth to a healthy baby boy named Oscar.

As with most illness, it was a confluence of events and stressors that led to my second time on an elemental diet. Until I weaned him from night nursing at 18 months, Oscar did not sleep more than three hours in a row, so neither did I. We also went to Singapore when Oscar was eight weeks old, for six months. However, when we came back to Vancouver, the new condo we had bought was far behind its construction schedule. So we then spent the next five and a half months travelling around England, Hawaii and Arizona, living out of suitcases. In addition, Oscar has a voracious appetite (and high metabolism) so he breastfed full feeds about ten times a day. Combined together, the stress of transatlantic flights, no home, no routines for the baby, all the varied adjustments involved for new parents, and the severe extended sleep deprivation eventually became too much for me.

I gradually lost weight until I was 115 lbs and then I took a new calcium/magnesium supplement I'd bought that also contained something called Betaine HCL (Hydrochloride). About eight hours later, my colon started bleeding. After wracking my brain to try and figure out what could have triggered the bleeding, I finally remembered the mystery ingredient and looked it up in one of my encyclopaedias. There I discovered that Betaine is something that stimulates the production of stomach acid. It should never be used by someone with ulcers and even people with normal digestive systems should start at a very low dose and stop if they experience any discomfort. Obviously, in a digestive system as sensitive as mine, that's all it took to trigger the bleeding and as I was so run down I knew the situation could deteriorate quite quickly.

I've found that you can use all kinds of herbal supplements to prop yourself up and keep going, but when your body becomes too run down and malnourished it loses the ability to heal itself. So even though you give it the tools, your body has no energy or resources left to utilize those tools. Although the bleeding wasn't anywhere near the haemorrhaging I experienced prior to the first time I went on an elemental diet, I didn't want to risk it escalating to that point, so I immediately went on an elemental diet after three days of passing blood, ranging from about 3 tbsp. - 1/4 cup per bowel movement, with small blood clots the second and third day.

The good news is that I was also nowhere near as ill and run down as I was the first time round, so although my bleeding had completely stopped by day four, I remained on the diet exclusively for two weeks. I then continued drinking a few shakes a day for an additional ten days as I gradually reintroduced normal food. I also didn't feel the need to gain weight as quickly as I did the first time, so I only consumed six shakes per day. At the end of two weeks I'd gained seven pounds and by the time I was fully back on regular food, I'd gained a total of 14 pounds. When I feel I need it, I have a shake in the morning as it's a great nutritional boost and an excellent way to take all my supplements in an easily digestible form. During my first pregnancy, I had a shake every morning with all the supplements and flax oil added as it's a wonderful way to ensure excellent health for both yourself and the baby.

However, a word of caution to women: The IBD Remission Diet is such a great rejuvenator of health that your fertility will also become very healthy and robust, so be very careful if you don't want to get pregnant! I got pregnant again, with my second child, two months after my second time on the IBD Remission Diet - in spite of using birth control! However, if you want to have kids, whether you're male or female, this diet will take your body (and hence your genetic material) to a new level of health, giving you the best chance of producing a healthy fetus. Studies have shown that the mother's nutritional status while the baby is in utero determines the health of the child up to 17 years later. I drank a shake containing all the supplements and flax oil 2-3 times/week throughout my second pregnancy as well. I am sure (along with a healthy, mostly organic diet and regular exercise) it's one of the principle reasons my children are so healthy. Oh yes, and I also don't degrade their immune systems with vaccinations. For more information on this, go to www.caramal.com (click on *Articles by Jini*) for my article on the short and long-term consequences of vaccination.

I haven't included any specific instructions in this book regarding when to consult your doctor and/or how to integrate drug therapy with the IBD Remission Diet, as I leave each of you free to do what you feel is best for your body. I included an entire chapter on my opinion on medical/pharmaceutical protocols in my first book, *LISTEN TO YOUR GUT* (www.caramal.com), so I won't repeat any of that here. If you wish, you can mix drugs (like Asacol, Prednisone, Salazopyrin, etc.) with the IBD Remission Diet; just give your doctor a full list of the supplements you're adding to the shakes so he/she is informed. In my opinion though, it's much better to wean yourself off your drugs before starting the Diet and give your body the full chance to restore its natural balance. If you're simultaneously taking immune suppressant drugs (like Prednisone, Imuran, etc.) whilst on the program I really don't know what results you'll have and how much you'll benefit. But again, you must do what you feel is safe and comfortable for yourself.

Both times I went on an elemental diet I consumed a variety of specifically chosen supplements as well as the nutritional shakes, and followed this with full-spectrum probiotics (good bacteria for both the small and large intestine). Therefore, I didn't just restore my weight but restored myself to great health as well. For me, health equals freedom. The freedom to eat what I want, to travel and have adventures, and to have enough energy to share joy and good times with my family and friends - the freedom to enjoy all the wonderful things that life and relationships have to offer. From the bottom of my heart, I wish for you this same joy and freedom.

TAKE ACTION

List contributing factors (or a spiral of events) that led up to your last flare:

_____

_____

_____

_____

_____

_____

_____

_____

_____

_____

_____

_____

_____

What are some things you could have done to halt or lessen the impact of these events? Use this knowledge to prevent a similar pattern/progression from occurring next time:

_____

_____

_____

_____

_____

_____

_____

_____

_____

_____

_____

_____

_____

If you were healthy, what are some of the things you'd like to do/accomplish with your newfound state of health:

_____

_____

_____

_____

_____

_____

_____

_____

_____

_____

_____

_____

_____

2

THE ELEMENTAL DIET

*Life affords no higher pleasure than that of
surmounting difficulties,
passing from one step of success to another,
forming new wishes and seeing them gratified.*
Samuel Johnson

A N ELEMENTAL DIET is one in which everything you consume - protein, carbohydrate, fat, vitamins, minerals, etc. - is in a completely pre-digested, liquid form. As a result, your body receives all the nutrients it needs with very minimal digestion required. Because everything is pre-digested, the nutrients are absorbed very quickly and your digestive system is given a chance to rest and heal. Also, because everything is pre-digested and completely absorbed, there is no undigested matter passing into the colon. This provides the colon with something doctors call 'bowel rest'. My gastroenterologist, who has a practice of about 600 patients with IBD, informed me that using an elemental diet to provide complete bowel rest results in disease remission as often as Prednisone (steroids). If you have ulceration, bleeding, fistulas, or fissures in your colon, every time you eat and have a bowel movement, the wounds are irritated and if they've started to clot or heal, the wounds will often be re-opened. An elemental diet provides the colon with the rest necessary to heal its wounds unhindered and the only fecal matter you pass is liquid, so anal and rectal fissures and fistulas also get the opportunity to heal undisturbed.

Another key result of having no undigested matter in the colon (and some parts of the small intestine) is that the resident bacterial population then has nothing to eat and will gradually starve to death and be excreted. This clearing of the bacterial flora in the colon is a major benefit of following the IBD Remission Diet. While the exact cause of Inflammatory Bowel Disease is not known, many theorise that a key causative factor is the overgrowth of bad bacteria in the intestine. This leads to 'Leaky Gut Syndrome', where undigested particles of food pass through the damaged intestinal lining directly into the bloodstream, where they trigger allergic reactions and immune system response. An elemental diet will starve off all these bad (and good) bacteria and the supplementation program will help your body heal the damaged intestinal wall and mucosal lining. Then, when you start eating regular food again, you supplement with probiotics (good bacteria) and re-populate your intestine with good bacteria that will help maintain intestinal health and control any bad bacteria that are later ingested.

Another key benefit of following the IBD Remission Diet is that it provides an ideal vehicle with which to consume large amounts of healing supplements in easily absorbable, liquid form. Swallowing 15 gelcaps, tablets, and capsules (for example) throughout the day for an extended period can be quite difficult and the absorption of these shellacked and capsulated products is not ideal. Emptying all those supplements into several good-tasting shakes and drinking them down is much easier, absorption is improved, and you're more likely to stick with it for the duration. As you'll see in Chapter Three, the supplements suggested have been chosen specifically to heal the mucosal lining of the intestine, reduce inflammation, repair tissue damage, support enzyme production and hormonal pathways, facilitate optimal cellular function, and balance the immune system. This provides your body with an extended healing spa where all aspects of digestive healing are supported simultaneously; and as the whole body is inter-linked, you may find that other health issues are also resolved during this time.

Many people with IBD (Inflammatory Bowel Disease) also suffer from malnutrition due to inadequate digestion, low absorption of nutrients, and lack of appetite - when everything you eat makes you feel sick or results in pain you quickly lose your appetite! The IBD Remission Diet is a fantastic way to resolve malnutrition and gain some solid weight (muscle, not fat) quickly. Because everything you consume is pre-digested, there is very little digestion required and the nutrients are absorbed rapidly. And because everything is in liquid form, it's easy to consume a large number of calories per day, so you can gain weight more quickly than if you were eating normal food. Also, even though your food is all in liquid form, you will not feel hungry on the elemental diet (as long as you're consuming an adequate number of calories for your body). In fact, some people who've followed the IBD Remission Diet have even been reluctant to go back to eating regular food - they loved the taste of the shakes, felt really good energy (not hungry at all) and very much enjoyed the break from shopping, meal planning, cooking and cleaning the kitchen! I also strongly advise that you start an exercise program - ideally weight training/body building - at the appropriate time to further encourage muscle growth and development. I'll go more into detail on this in Chapter Five.

If you stay on the IBD Remission Diet for two weeks or longer, you'll also experience the benefits of a natural, gradual and gentle detoxification. Your cells, organs and digestive system will release and flush toxins, old waste and any impacted fecal matter. Again, if you get pregnant following the IBD Remission Diet, you're more likely to have a nausea-free pregnancy due to the detoxification of your liver and cells. This detoxification is facilitated not only by the liquid, pre-digested diet, but also by the specific supplements that support liver, digestive, and cellular health.

Within a day or two of beginning the elemental diet, you'll pass only liquid feces and your bowel movements may be a strange color or look weird to you. All natural coloring agents used in the elemental shakes will go straight through to your bowel movements and you will also be flushing toxins and possibly experiencing 'bile purges' from your gall bladder - which may add up to very strange looking fecal matter. As well, don't be surprised if your bowel movements become very urgent. Liquid fecal matter is usually explosive and hard to hold in. You can use the Bowel Control technique in Chapter Seven of my book, *LISTEN TO YOUR GUT*, or just make sure you stay near a bathroom when necessary.

The main difficulty in following a liquid, elemental diet is simply one of food/taste deprivation. It is very hard to go for days and weeks without being able to eat normally and having to say 'no' to nearly every yummy thing around you. Of course, the sicker you are, the easier it is to maintain this kind of discipline as your motivation is really high! Therefore, I have included recipes and suggestions for as much variety as is allowed on this type of diet. If you just drink sweet shakes all the time, your appetite will not be very stimulated and you'll hit 'taste fatigue' pretty quickly. This makes it hard to consume the number of calories required for weight gain, or even weight maintenance. Therefore, I've included recipes for all kinds of really tasty meat, vegetable and mushroom broths that provide a 'salty' alternative to the sweet taste of the shakes. Alternating sweet and salty tastes keeps your palate interested and your appetite stimulated. I've also included recipes for homemade jello, and there are certain types of gummy bears and chewing gum that fit the elemental parameters and these are included also. It's good to have something to chew on occasionally as your teeth and gums need some stimulation and exercise as well during this period.

How Long Should I Stay On The Elemental Diet?

The first time I went on an elemental diet, I followed it for seven weeks. The second time, I only needed to stay on it for two weeks. The length of time you choose to remain on an elemental diet should be guided by three factors: The severity of your illness when you first begin, the status of your ongoing symptoms as the diet progresses, and most importantly, your intuition.

Your body knows exactly what it needs and when it needs it. All you have to do is ask, and then honor the wisdom received by acting on it. Accessing your body's wisdom is very simple. Lie or sit somewhere quietly, wherever you feel most relaxed - it may be in your bed, your living room, at the beach or in the forest, or in the bathtub with some candles lit. Do some deep breathing for a while to relax your body and your mind. When your limbs feel heavy and you maybe feel a little sleepy, place your hand on your belly and ask your colon/digestive system how long it needs you to stay on the elemental diet. If you're not used to using your intuition, or asking your body for guidance, the feeling you get may be quite vague or faint. Don't worry about that, no matter how 'iffy' the first answer or impression feels, act on it and stick to it. If you're not used to using your intuition, you may get several answers/feelings/impressions as your conscious, doubting and nervous mind interferes. Stick with the *first* answer or feeling and ignore the rest. The more often you use your intuition - and using it involves acting on the answers, not just asking the questions - the stronger it will become.

Now let's say your intuition tells you, 'four weeks', so you begin the elemental diet with the intention of sticking to it for four weeks. But, at week number two you're feeling really good and you start to think, "Hey, maybe I don't need to stay on it the full four weeks…" - don't give in to these feelings! You asked your body and your body told you what it needed and it's best that you honor your body by following through. Of course, if your feelings are very strong, then relax yourself again (as described above) and ask your body for further instructions.

Another guideline to help you determine the duration of your elemental diet is your state of illness at the outset. In my opinion, if you're experiencing any of the following, then you should go on the diet for at least six weeks:

- Steady intestinal bleeding or haemorrhaging.
- Moderate to severe malnutrition, as determined by your albumin levels (your doctor can order a blood test to check this), or a skeletal appearance.
- The presence of fistulas.
- Your doctor suggesting strongly that you undergo surgery.

If you've been haemorrhaging, you may experience minimal bleeding - a few small traces or streaks of blood in the stool or on the toilet paper - throughout the diet. Don't worry about this, it can be healed later using the herbal remedies described in my first book, *LISTEN TO YOUR GUT* (www.caramal.com), although, if you prefer, you can certainly remain on the elemental diet until all the bleeding is completely eradicated. Complete healing of severe conditions like fistulas may require you to stay on the elemental diet for up to three months, but for most serious conditions six weeks should be sufficient. If you're experiencing only sporadic intestinal bleeding, then four to six weeks on the elemental diet should be sufficient to heal and stop the bleeding - however, you may wish to err on the side of caution here and do the full six weeks.

If you're not experiencing any bleeding or other serious symptoms, but you'd just like to revamp and clear up an assortment of minor symptoms like bloating, gas, pain upon eating, diarrhea, spastic bowel, severe heartburn, etc, then three to four weeks should be sufficient. If you want to use the IBD Remission Diet primarily to test for food allergies, you'll need to go on the elemental diet for approximately 10 - 14 days, or however long it takes to clear up most of your symptoms. Make sure you add all the recommended supplements to the shakes as well. Two weeks is also a sufficient length of time if you're already doing quite well but just want to purify/detoxify your body and balance immune system functioning.

Monitoring your symptoms whilst on the elemental diet can provide you with another guideline of how long to remain on it. Make a list of the symptoms you wish to heal whilst on the diet and then stay on it for at least one to two more weeks after all of your symptoms have cleared. This is a good way of really establishing the healing that has taken place. The last thing you want is to have your symptoms return as soon as you start eating food and then have to go back on the diet again for another three to six weeks. I really encourage you to err on the side of caution here as it's much easier to just stay on the diet a bit longer than to stop, eat normal food for a while, and then have to start all over back on the elemental diet again. My second time on an elemental diet (duration two weeks) happened to occur over the Christmas season - talk about torture! I had to sit there with all this incredible food and endless snacks and chocolate around everywhere and not have a single bite! Even though I had stopped bleeding before Christmas Day, it just wasn't worth the risk for day or two of delicious food. At times like these, you've got to put things in perspective. Count up the number of Christmases (or birthdays, etc.) you have left in your life, then you'll realise that giving up one for your body and long-term health is not asking too much.

When I initially discussed elemental diet durations with my gastroenterologist, he gave me the standard that he uses. He advises patients to go on the elemental diet for either three or six weeks. However, he cautioned, if you only go on it for three weeks and then your symptoms return, you'll need to go back on it for the full six weeks (nine weeks total). Simply going back on the elemental diet for an additional three weeks is not good enough as the body needs to heal in an uninterrupted manner. Therefore, my first time on the elemental diet I decided to stay on it for seven weeks just to be sure!

In many cases, regardless of length of time on the elemental diet, when you begin the transition to normal food you may see traces of blood in your stool or on the toilet paper. This can occur as your rectum and anus adjust to the larger, firmer stool, which sometimes causes minor rectal/anal fissures. These fissures will usually just heal themselves within a month or two, or you can order effective herbal suppositories called FissureHeal (www.fissureheal.com) to speed the healing considerably. I've used FissureHeal suppositories to heal both a minor and severe anal fissure and they work really well. They contain Slippery Elm, Marshmallow Root, Comfrey Root and Cocoa Butter, and they're also ultra-thin so can be easily inserted into even the most sore and traumatized rectum. See Appendix A for further order details. Of course, if you already have anal/rectal fissures that need healing, you can use the FissureHeal suppositories whilst on the elemental diet, or at any other time. Insert them at night - or whenever you're likely to have your longest stretch without a bowel movement - so your rectum has the maximum amount of time to heal undisturbed.

Don't be surprised if your symptoms actually worsen during the first 3-4 days on the diet. As the body cleanses and releases toxins, symptoms can temporarily worsen, or they may also be a result of you withdrawing from addictive substances like caffeine. Many people take time off work during this period and treat the process like a healing vacation, getting plenty of rest, massage, meditating, etc. It also helps to be off work as, dependent upon your required daily caloric intake, you may have to mix up an elemental shake every 2-3 hours. If you want to use this as a time to simultaneously put on some weight, then you'll need to consume between 2500-4000 calories per day, depending on how much weight you want to gain and how quickly you want to do it. I used the IBD Remission Diet on its own to go from 104 pounds to 125 pounds in only five weeks.

I consumed 3500-3700 calories per day, which meant I had to eat every one and a half to two hours, from morning until bedtime. This may be too fast and too intense for many people, so again, only do what feels right for your body.

You may also have a concern about the cost involved in following the IBD Remission Diet. This can indeed be an expensive endeavour. The first time I went on an elemental diet - for seven weeks - the total cost, including supplements was about US$2900.00. Fortunately for you, buying Absorb Plus (the elemental shake product I recommend) is much cheaper than buying all the ingredients separately and mixing them together the way I had to at that time. But it will still probably cost you about US$1000.00-1800.00 for a six week stint on the IBD Remission Diet. Again, although that may seem expensive, it helps to put it in perspective. The cost is still less than you'd spend on a two week vacation and look at what you get in return. In return for my seven weeks on the elemental diet I completely healed a severely hemorrhaging colon, restored myself from severe malnutrition and anemia to perfect health, avoided surgery, drugs and hospital visits, got pregnant, had a wonderful pregnancy and a very healthy child, and had the level of health and strength needed to get me through two very stressful years following of severe sleep deprivation, constant breastfeeding and moving halfway round the world and back again! My second, two week stint on the elemental diet, cost me a total of US$600 and in return I got another healthy pregnancy, healthy baby, and years following of strength, health and vitality. When you look at it in those terms, it's actually very cheap and the sacrifice small compared to the returns!

Also, make sure you check with your health insurance company about getting partial or total coverage for the cost of Absorb Plus. This may be possible if you get a letter from your doctor stating that an elemental diet is his/her recommended course of treatment. Likewise, in some countries, depending on the laws, you may be able to deduct the partial or full cost of Absorb Plus (or whatever elemental products you use) from your income tax return.

ELEMENTAL FOODS

It's necessary to consume a balanced diet of protein, fat, and carbohydrates whilst on the IBD Remission Diet. Following are the allowable forms of each nutrient in elemental form and my recommendations for each:

Protein

- Hydrolyzed whey protein (specifically called whey protein isolate)
- Hydrolyzed soy protein (soy protein isolate)
- Hydrolyzed rice protein

I strongly recommend you use whey protein if at all possible as it has the highest bioavailability of all the forms of hydrolyzed protein. This means your body can absorb and utilise more of it, resulting in more muscle, much faster than with any of the other forms of protein. Make sure the whey protein has been extracted from the milk using a cold, ion-exchange, cross-flow membrane extraction method, as heat or chemical extraction methods de-nature the protein. Most people who have an allergy or intolerance to cow's milk are allergic to either the lactose (a milk sugar), or a dominant milk protein called casein. If you're lactose intolerant, whey protein isolate is most likely safe for you as usually 99.8% of the lactose has been removed. If you're allergic to milk protein, then you will probably still be able to use whey protein isolate, because in certain brands of whey protein isolate (check the label), all of the casein has been removed too. Do not purchase whey protein concentrate as this is not the same as whey protein isolate.

Aside from the strong taste, I don't like using soy protein because it depresses thyroid function, blocks mineral absorption, contains a lot of estrogen, and the manufacturing process for soy protein (and soy milk) renders it somewhat toxic. In addition, it's less bio-available to the body than whey protein, so you have to consume more of it to get the same results. Rice protein has none of the damaging effects of soy protein, but it's even less bio-available than soy. Still, for that extremely small percentage of you who are allergic to whey protein, you'll have to go with one or the other and I'll leave it up to you to make that decision. Consult with your naturopathic physician for further guidance. Keep in mind that most stores will let you return a product if you don't like the taste, so if you need to experiment, keep your receipt!

Carbohydrates

- Maltodextrin
- Fructose
- Glucose
- Dextrose

Again, all your carbohydrates must be pre-digested so even regular sugar or honey are not allowed.

Fat

- Cold-pressed Flax oil
- Udo's Choice Perfected Oil Blend
- Cold-pressed Hemp seed oil
- Cold-pressed Safflower oil
- Cold-pressed Virgin or Extra-Virgin Olive oil
- Certified Organic Butter

I recommend you use either flax oil or Udo's Choice Perfected Oil Blend in the shakes as their taste is quite mild and unobtrusive - in addition to the beneficial, anti-inflammatory Omega-3 essential fatty acids they contain. Flax oil is a very delicate, unstable oil, so make sure you only buy an organic, cold-pressed brand that's been kept in the refrigerator (Spectrum Naturals is the best brand). Be sure to buy a small bottle and keep it refrigerated, use it up within 4-6 weeks of opening so it doesn't start to oxidize (become rancid) and irritate your gut. If you've been haemorrhaging or are very sensitive to oil, then keep your bottle of flax oil in the freezer (it doesn't solidify completely) and squeeze it out as needed - this reduces the oxidation by 95%. If you find you're still sensitive to flax oil, then try the Udo's Oil - you may find it better tolerated. Also, if you're going to buy a brand of flax oil other than Spectrum Naturals, contact the company to ascertain whether they cold-pasteurize the oil. If they don't and you're highly sensitive, you may react to the tiny mold spores or parasites that may be present in oil that hasn't been cold-pasteurized.

Depending on your level of health (liver function, antioxidant capability, etc.) you'll be able to consume more or less oil. So let your body and your symptoms be your guide to find the level of supplementation that's right for your body. You can also use hemp oil, but the taste is quite strong so you may not like it. You may want to use flax oil in one shake, then Udo's in the next, and so on throughout the day. The Udo's is more expensive though, so if cost is an issue, then just use the flax oil. If you're completely intolerant of any liquid oils, then take enteric-coated capsules of either flax oil, or fish oil (make sure the company tests for fish oil toxicity though). The other oils and butter can be used for frying the meats and mushrooms in when you make your broths (recipes to follow).

Other Allowables
- Clear fruit juices
- Popsicles made from clear fruit juices
- Jello made from clear fruit juice and gelatin
- Clear soup broths
- Clear, organic herbal teas (caffeine-free only, can be sweetened with Stevia or fructose if you wish)
- Certain brands of gummy bears (no more than 10 per day)
- Wrigley's brand regular Spearmint or Juicy Fruit chewing gum (maximum 5 sticks per day)

Make sure all fruit juices are fresh (not from concentrate) with no additives like sugar, color, or preservatives. Obviously, certified organic fruit juice is preferable - make sure it's see-through clear with no clouding. Juice from a home or commercial juicer is not allowed as there's too much pulp residue in the juice. To make fruit juice popsicles, just buy a popsicle mold from a housewares store, pour in the clear juice of your choice (dilute a bit with water if you prefer) add the popsicle sticks/tops and then freeze. See the recipe section for instructions on making the jello and soup broths. If you don't want to make your own broths, you can use canned or packaged, but make sure they're see-through clear and certified organic, with no added thickeners, pureed vegetables, etc. Look for gummy bears made primarily from fruit juice, with no artificial flavors, sweeteners, colors or preservatives and using only the allowable sugars and gelatin listed above - again, don't consume more than ten per day. If a soup or juice looks slightly opaque and you're not sure whether it's safe or not, either phone the manufacturer directly to find out what's in it or how they make it, or just avoid it. You will not experience proper clearing of your bacterial flora if you have any undigested food matter passing into your colon for the bacteria to eat and stay alive on. For this reason, it's better to err on the side of caution.

If you're desperate to have something to chew on, you can chew meat as long as you don't swallow anything and spit the pieces out once the flavor's gone. For myself, I find there's nothing like the flavor of a good piece of steak fat! I buy a piece of organic sirloin steak with the fat intact. I pan fry it in butter, a little garlic and salt and then cut off the strip of fat leaving a ½ inch of meat intact along the side. I brown the fat until it's crispy on the outside and then I savour each bite. If you do this, as you chew, some of the fat will turn liquid and it's okay to swallow that, but be sure and spit the rest out. I then give the remaining sirloin steak to someone else to eat, or use it to make steak broth (see recipe section). You can also get your butcher to save you the strips of fat when he trims the meat for packaging and just buy that. But make sure it's organic meat, as an animal's toxins and hormones are stored in its fat and it would be very unhealthy to eat regular (non-organic) steak fat. Of course, for some people, chewing something tasty and not being able to swallow it would feel more like torture and make it more difficult to stick with the diet. Do what works for you.

MIXING THE ELEMENTAL SHAKES

These shakes will provide all your nutrition and required calories on the IBD Remission Diet. The other items like broths, jello and gummy bears are great for variety but provide only minimal calories. Although the home-made soup broths do provide fantastic nutrition (see recipe section) their caloric content is still very low. You can mix up your own shakes as I had to, if you prefer, and I will provide instructions for that. However, there is also now a product available that contains all the elemental nutrients you need together in one formula - all you have to add is water and flax oil. And I should know, because I created it! One of the founders of a health product company called Imix Naturals Inc., asked me to put together the formula after reading my book, *LISTEN TO YOUR GUT.* I agreed and they called the resulting product Absorb Plus. It contains whey protein, maltodextrin, fructose, glucose, a complete vitamin/mineral profile and 10 highly beneficial amino acids, including one gram of L-Glutamine per serving. You'll see the importance of L-Glutamine in Chapter Three. It's all natural - no artificial flavors, sweeteners, or preservatives - and comes in Chocolate Royale, French Vanilla or Mixed Berry flavor. I took a long time to get the flavoring right and, in my opinion, Absorb Plus tastes much better than anything else out there. Well, I leave it up to you, do your own research and taste testing and you be the judge. Sometimes the company will provide free samples, so check if that's available. Order details for Absorb Plus are in Appendix A, or you can check it out on their website at www.absorbplus.com.

Although Absorb Plus (and other whey protein products) is available in three different flavors, if you have a sensitivity to chocolate it's best to still avoid it, or keep it to a minimum whilst on the elemental diet. See the Recipe section in Chapter Three for ways you may be able to incorporate chocolate even though you're sensitive to it - if you really love the taste. However, if your sensitivity is to caffeine, keep in mind that each serving of Absorb Plus Chocolate Royale contains only .008 mg. of caffeine per serving. By comparison, a cup of coffee contains 125-185 mg., a cup of tea 45-60 mg. and a cup of green tea 15-20 mg. of caffeine.

If you prefer to mix up your own shakes (but research it first as it will probably be more expensive than just buying Absorb Plus and the taste won't be very good), here's what you need to get:

- Ion-exchange, cold, cross-flow membrane extracted whey protein with no artificial sweeteners, colors or flavors (splenda/sucralose, acesulfame-K, and aspartame are all artificial sweeteners and not allowed). Or, if you're allergic to whey, a hydrolyzed protein substitute like soy or brown rice, or goat whey protein.

- A pre-digested carbohydrate product containing only maltodextrin, fructose, glucose or dextrose. Make sure the maltodextrin is the major component in the mix (ideally 75% or higher).

- A full-spectrum complete multi-vitamin and multi-mineral. You may need to purchase several different products to get a full spectrum of both major and trace minerals and vitamins.

- It would be nice to include an array of amino acids. Allergy Research Corp. makes a product at this time called Free Aminos, but if you can't find it, just make sure to get some L-Glutamine, which is the primary nutrient for the intestinal wall and mucosal lining.

- If you need additional sweetness, you can use either fructose or white stevia powder or liquid (an herb 200-300 times sweeter than table sugar).

Basic Shake Mixture if Not Using Absorb Plus

- 25 grams of whey protein (or protein alternate)
- 50 grams of carbohydrate mix
- 1 capsule of multi-vitamin/mineral
- 1 gram of L-Glutamine
- 2 grams total of mixed amino acids in free-form

This will provide you with your basic single serving shake mixture, so use this wherever you see 'one serving of Absorb Plus' called for.

I used to give brand name recommendations for the whey protein and carbohydrate components, but I've found that sports supplement companies change brands and formulas quite often, so it can be misleading. Your health store should be able to find you what you need and if you have difficulty finding the carbohydrate component, then check out www.nutramed.com, but make sure the product contains no oil. If it contains vitamins, minerals and amino acids then delete the duplicated items from the Basic Shake Mixture recipe above. Obviously, if you're truly allergic to whey protein, you can substitute soy or rice protein but you'll have to consume more of it to gain/maintain the same amount of weight. If you substitute just free-form amino acids for the protein component, this will be good for your health but you won't be able to gain any weight on it. In order for protein to be used for muscle fibre it needs to have a least a di-peptide bond for uptake and utilisation - which free-form amino acids do not. Keep checking periodically with the company that makes Absorb Plus though (www.imixnaturals.com), as I know they're currently working on an all-natural, vegetable protein elemental diet product.

This Basic Shake Mixture then needs to be added to the following ingredients (in place of Absorb Plus) to form the standard Elemental Shake Recipe you'll be using throughout the IBD Remission Diet. Obviously, if you choose to purchase Absorb Plus, you can ignore all the information above and just start here:

IBD Remission Diet Elemental Shake Recipe

1. Pour 1 cup (8 oz) of cold or room-temperature spring or filtered water into a blender

2. Add 1 serving of Absorb Plus (100 grams/4 level scoops)

3. Add the supplements of your choice (see Chapter Three)

4. Add 1 tsp. - 1 tbsp. of organic flax or Udo's oil (according to tolerance)

5. Whip on high speed for 10-15 seconds

6. Pour into a glass over ice and drink through a straw.

Drink the shake slowly; take at least 15-30 minutes to consume it. You may want to follow each shake with 1 glass of spring or filtered water, as the maltodextrin can absorb a lot of liquid. If you feel a bit nauseous, then drink the shake more slowly, or lower the oil content, or drink water between shakes. Also keep in mind that this is a new food source so give your body some time to adjust to it. You may want to start with just 2-3 shakes per day and gradually increase from there to the 5-8 shakes per day you'll probably need.

It's best if you can add one tablespoon of organic flax or Udo's oil per shake. If you have a fat intolerance problem, then just start with one teaspoon (or less) and gradually work up to one tablespoon. Usually people with a 'fat intolerance' problem are intolerant of hydrogenated fat, which contains damaging trans-fatty acids (commercial vegetable oils, margarine, the fat in deep fried foods and processed foods, etc.). Cold-pressed flax oil is not hydrogenated and is absorbed very quickly, and even people with a marked 'fat-intolerance' have no problem with it. Flax oil also contains high levels of Omega-3, which is a powerful anti-inflammatory and has been used solely in double-blind, placebo controlled studies to induce remission in patients with Crohn's Disease (*The New England Journal of Medicine, June 13, 1996*). If you find you can't tolerate adding liquid flax oil to the shakes (even when you've kept your bottle of flax oil in the freezer), then take it in enteric-coated capsules - some people argue that as the capsules protect completely against oxidation, they are better tolerated by people with high sensitivities (due to a weakened liver or poor antioxidant defense, etc). A pristine source of fish oil (make sure the company tests for toxicity) in enteric-coated capsules will also give you all the benefits of the Omega-3s and other Essential Fatty Acids. Take as many of these enteric-coated capsules as you can tolerate, to a maximum of 15 per day. Aside from their anti-inflammatory properties, the Essential Fatty Acids (EFAs) contained in flax oil also benefit the body in the following ways, they:

- are a ready source of energy
- provide insulation for your body against heat loss
- prevent your skin from drying or flaking

- are a cushion for your tissues and organs
- stimulate production of "prostaglandin" families - hormones necessary for cell-to-cell biochemical functions such as energy metabolism, cardiovascular and immune system health.

For the Udo's Choice Perfected Oil Blend, see their product literature (or www.udoerasmus.com) for a full description of all the wonderful oils in it and why they're so beneficial for your body. You can safely supplement up to 8 tablespoons per day of flax or Udo's oil and a good maintenance dose, once you're off the elemental diet, is 1-2 tablespoons per day or as often as you feel you need it.

HOW MANY SHAKES PER DAY SHOULD I DRINK?

The number of shakes per day that you should consume depends on your existing weight, how much weight you want to gain, and how much oil you're adding per shake. You need to take two factors into account when calculating the number of shakes that's right for you: Amount of protein and calorie count. Ideally, you want to add as much oil as you can tolerate per shake because aside from its health benefits, adding oil helps to increase the calorie count per shake. A 100 gram serving of Absorb Plus contains roughly 370 calories per serving (each flavor has a slightly different calorie count: Vanilla is 365 calories, Berry is 370 and Chocolate is 374 calories). One teaspoon of flax oil is 40 calories and one tablespoon of flax oil is 120 calories. The final calorie count of your shake depends on how much flax oil you add so, as I said, add as much as you can, up to your personal tolerance level.

Calculating Your Daily Protein Allowance

If you want to maintain your existing weight, you need a minimum of one gram of protein per one kilogram of body weight each day. However, since you're on an elemental diet and you can't get carbohydrates from a separate source (unless you buy maltodextrin on its own), you also need to make sure your calorie count is high enough to maintain your existing weight as well (see the next section). It's okay to consume more whey protein than your body actually needs, as you'll just excrete it in urine.

To calculate your weight in kilograms, take your weight in pounds and divide it by 2.2 (1 kg = 2.2 lbs). Suppose you weigh 50 kilograms: To maintain your existing weight you must consume at least 50 grams of protein per day. However, if you want to gain weight, then you need to consume three grams of protein for every kilogram of body weight. So, if you weigh 50 kg, you need to consume 150 grams of protein per day. Keep in mind that as your body weight increases, you will need to increase the amount of protein accordingly if you want to keep on gaining weight.

Calculating Your Daily Caloric Needs

The number of calories you need just to maintain your existing weight varies according to your activity level. If you're a sedentary person, you need 13 calories per pound to maintain your existing weight. If you're moderately active, you need to consume 15 calories per pound, and if you're extremely active, you need 17 calories per pound to maintain your existing weight. Therefore, if you're a sedentary person weighing 100 pounds, you need to consume 1300 calories per day just to maintain that weight.

It takes 3000 calories to create one pound of body weight. Therefore, in addition to the number of calories needed to maintain your existing weight, you need to consume 3000 extra calories for every pound you want to gain. For example, if you're a sedentary person weighing 100 pounds and you consume 2000 calories per day, you'll gain weight at a moderate pace (about one pound every five days). If you consume 3000 calories per day, you'll gain weight quickly (about one pound every two days). It really depends on what your goals are - how much weight you want to gain and how quickly.

So, in addition to calculating your protein allowance for the day, you also have to figure out your caloric requirements and then try to meld the two together to come up with how many shakes you need to consume each day. Absorb Plus is 370 calories with 27 grams of protein (including the amino acids) per serving. If you add 1 table-spoon of flax oil per shake, you bring the calorie count up to 490 per shake. Let's say you weigh 100 pounds and you want to just maintain your weight. You will only require two servings of Absorb Plus to meet your protein requirement for the day. However, two servings of Absorb Plus (with 1 tbsp. flax oil per shake) will only give you 980 calories for the day, and you need 1300 calories to maintain your weight at 100 pounds. So in this case, you'll need to consume three servings of Absorb Plus per day to maintain your weight.

Your Current Weight pounds / kg.	Shakes per Day to Maintain Current Weight	Shakes per Day to Gain Weight
95 pounds / 43 kg.	3 shakes	4 - 5 shakes
110 pounds / 50 kg.	3.5 shakes	5 shakes
125 pounds / 57 kg.	4 shakes	6 shakes
140 pounds / 64 kg.	4.5 shakes	7 shakes

INABILITY TO GAIN WEIGHT

If you're consuming a sufficient number of calories and grams of protein per day and you're still not gaining weight, then book an appointment with a naturopath who's experienced with hormones. Chronic stress, illness and pharmaceutical drugs (especially steroids) can really mess up your adrenal gland and hormone levels and result in all kinds of problems from impaired thyroid function to a deficit or surplus of key hormones involved in weight regulation. If you've been on prescription steroids (eg. Prednisone) or other immune suppressant drugs (eg. Imuran), or birth control pills, you definitely need to have your thyroid and hormone levels checked. However, as hormonal health is still a relatively new field you need to find a physician (MD or ND) who specializes in hormones and has lots of experience reading and interpreting hormone tests combined with symptom profiles.

I had two doctors (an MD and an ND) tell me my hormone levels were normal, when I knew intuitively there was something wrong with them. I was eating three meals plus two protein shakes per day and I was still losing weight. I was freezing cold all the time and even when I used a hot water bottle or bath to warm up, I wouldn't stay warm afterwards. I was very irritable and felt depressed many days and I was usually very tired. I finally found a doctor who specialized in hormone health and she ascertained that my thyroid was low, my cortisol levels very high, and my estrogen, progesterone and testosterone very all very low as well. I began supplementing with raw adrenal gland extract, thyroid extract, DHEA, and natural progesterone cream. From my second day of supplementation, I was no longer cold and I began gaining about three pounds per week. My mental/emotional symptoms also subsided very quickly and my energy increased proportionately.

If you're a woman over the age of twenty, I highly recommend you purchase a book called, *What Your Doctor May Not Tell You About Premenopause* by John R. Lee, MD and Jesse Hanley, MD. Don't let the title mislead you, this is the best book on hormonal imbalances I have read, and all the factors - from plastic food containers to synthetic clothing to emotional/lifestyle factors - that contribute to hormonal imbalance are covered. The book also goes into hormone testing and therapy in detail so it's an invaluable resource guide if you suspect your hormone levels are off, or that your adrenal or thyroid glands are not functioning properly. For men, there's a little booklet available in most health stores called *Natural Progesterone Cream: Safe and Natural Hormone Replacement* (A Keats Good Health Guide) by C. Norman Shealy, MD, PhD, that is helpful - particularly if you have, or your family has, a history of prostate gland problems.

Most hormonal supplements your naturopath prescribes can just be added to the shakes along with the rest of your supplements. DHEA is tasteless and raw adrenal extract is pretty bland as long as it doesn't have other substances added, raw thyroid extract (like

Armour Thyroid) is a very small pill that can be swallowed or chewed easily. Do not take synthetic hormones as they do not have the same holistic, supportive effect on the body - make sure all hormones and thyroid or adrenal supplements are 100% natural. You may also want to try homeopathic thyroid and adrenal support medicines. During my second pregnancy, I used a homeopathic formula that provided support for my thyroid, liver, spleen, pituitary, pancreas and adrenal and found it very effective. We monitored my thyroid levels (TSH) throughout my pregnancy with blood tests and the homeopathic remedy (along with good diet, nutritional supplements and exercise) resulted in consistent, marked improvement throughout the pregnancy. A hypothyroid can cause mental retardation in the fetus so it's not something you want to take chances with! Above all, if you suspect you have a hormonal imbalance the important thing is to find a doctor who specializes in hormones - an ordinary GP or ND (or gastroenterologist) will not be skilled enough to interpret your test results and symptoms accurately.

TAKE ACTION

How Long Should I Stay on the Elemental Diet?

1. List your symptoms here - all the symptoms you'd like to see resolved by following the IBD Remission Diet:

    _____

    _____

    _____

    _____

    _____

    _____

    _____

2. Perform the relaxation exercise and ask your own intuition how long you should remain on the diet:

    _____ weeks

3. Examine your answers above and combine with the guidelines given in this chapter for suggested length of time on the Diet (remember to err on the side of caution!). Therefore, you should remain on the Diet for:

    _____ weeks

How Many Shakes per Day Should I Drink?

To maintain your existing weight

First, figure out:
1. how many calories and
2. how much protein you need per day just to maintain your existing weight.

1. Current weight in pounds:____ x 15 = _____calories required

   Amount of flax oil you intend to add per shake
   (*40 calories per teaspoon, 120 calories per tablespoon*):_____

   Absorb Plus is approximately 370 calories per serving
   + _____flax oil calories = _____total calories per shake.

   Therefore:

   $$\frac{\text{calories required per day}}{\text{total calories per shake}} = \underline{\hspace{1cm}}\text{SHAKES PER DAY}$$

2. Current weight in pounds:_____ ÷ 2.2 = _____weight in kg

   Current weight in kg:____ x 1 = ____grams of protein required

   Absorb Plus contains 27 grams of protein per serving

   Therefore:

   $$\frac{\text{grams of protein needed per day}}{27} = \underline{\hspace{1cm}}\text{SHAKES PER DAY}$$

Now, based on your caloric and protein requirements (see 1. and 2.), how many Absorb Plus shakes do you need to drink per day just to maintain your existing weight (take whichever one is higher - if you drink more protein than you need, don't worry, you'll just pee it out):

_____ **shakes needed per day to maintain your existing weight.**

EXAMPLE: Charles weighs 160 lbs.

He needs 2400 calories (160 lbs x 15 = 2400) per day to maintain his weight. He's going to add 2 teaspoons of flax oil per shake, so each shake will be 450 calories (370 + 80 = 450). Therefore, based on his caloric needs, he needs to drink 6 shakes per day to maintain his weight (2400 ÷ 450= 5.33).

The second part of Charles' body requirements is his protein count. Charles weighs 72.7 kilograms (160 lbs ÷ 2.2 = 72.7 kg). Therefore, Charles needs 73 grams of protein per day to maintain his existing weight. Absorb Plus contains 27 grams of protein per serving, so he needs 3 Absorb Plus shakes per day to meet his protein requirement (73 ÷ 27 = 2.7). However, 3 shakes per day won't provide him with nearly enough calories, therefore, he still needs to drink 6 Absorb Plus shakes per day to meet his caloric requirements. **Therefore, Charles needs to drink 6 shakes per day just to maintain his existing weight.**

Important: If Charles could increase the amount of flax oil he adds per shake (to 1 tablespoon = 120 calories), he could then lower the number of servings of Absorb Plus required since the increased flax oil would help him make up his calorie requirement.

To gain weight

First, figure out:

    1. how many calories and

    2. how much protein you need per day to gain weight.

1.   Current weight in pounds:_____ x 15 = _____ calories
needed per day to maintain weight [A].

To add 1 pound of body weight requires consuming 3000 extra calories above your daily maintenance calories required. So:

    a. To gain weight **very quickly** (1 lb per day):
       Take [A] _____ + 3000 = _____ calories per day

    b. To gain weight **quite quickly** (0.5 lb per day):
       Take [A] _____ + 1500 = _____ calories per day

    c. To gain weight **reasonably quickly** (1 lb every 3 days):
       Take [A] _____ + 1000 = _____ calories per day

Amount of flax oil you intend to add per shake
(40 calories per teaspoon, 120 calories per tablespoon):_____

Absorb Plus is approximately 370 calories per serving
+ _____flax oil calories = _____total calories per shake.

Therefore:

$$\frac{\text{calories required per day [a,b or c]}}{\text{calories total per shake}} = \underline{\quad}\text{SHAKES PER DAY}$$

2.   Current weight in pounds:_____ ÷ 2.2 = _____weight in kg

Current weight in kg:____ x 3 = ____ grams of protein required

Absorb Plus contains 27 grams of protein per serving

Therefore:

$$\frac{\text{grams of protein needed per day}}{27} = \underline{\quad}\text{SHAKES PER DAY}$$

Now, based on your caloric and protein requirements (as calculated in 1. and 2.), how many Absorb Plus shakes do you need to drink per day to gain weight (take whichever one is higher - if you drink more protein than you need, don't worry, you'll just pee it out):

_____ shakes per day needed to gain weight.

VERY IMPORTANT: Make sure you re-do this calculation for every 10-15 pounds you gain. As your weight increases, your caloric needs will also increase, so you'll need to drink more shakes per day if you want to keep gaining weight.

EXAMPLE: Nina weighs 100 lbs.

She needs 1500 calories per day just to maintain her weight (100 x 15 = 1500). She wants to gain weight fairly quickly though (0.5 lb per day) so she'll need to consume 3000 calories per day to gain weight at her desired pace (1500 + 1500 = 3000). She's going to add 1 tablespoon of flax oil per shake, so each shake will be 490 calories (370 + 120 = 490). Therefore, based on her caloric needs, she needs to drink 6 shakes per day to gain weight (3000 ÷ 490 = 6.12).

The second part of Nina's body requirement is her protein count. Nina weighs 45.5 kilograms (100 ÷ 2.2 = 45.5 kg). Therefore, Nina needs to consume 136.5 grams of protein per day to gain weight (45.5 grams x 3 = 136.5). Absorb Plus contains 27 grams of protein per serving, so she needs to drink 5 Absorb Plus shakes per day just to meet her protein requirement (136.5 ÷ 27 = 5.05). However, 5 shakes per day won't provide her with enough calories, therefore, **she needs to drink 6 Absorb Plus shakes per day to meet her protein and calorie requirements and gain weight at her desired pace.**

Important: When Nina's weight reaches 110 lbs, she'll need to drink 6.5 shakes per day to continue to gain weight, and by the time she weighs 120 lbs, she'll need to drink 7 shakes per day to continue to gain weight at the same pace.

How Much Absorb Plus do I Need to Order?

Use your calculations (depending on whether you want to gain weight or just maintain your existing weight) and write down here the number of Absorb Plus shakes you need to drink per day.

_____

Each tub of Absorb Plus contains approximately 10 servings, so:
number of shakes you need to drink per day   _____
multiply by days you intend to stay on the diet   x _____
total shakes needed for entire duration   = _____

Then, take the total shakes needed:_____ ÷ 10 servings per tub = _____ number of tubs of Absorb Plus needed for the duration of the Diet.

*You'll also need to order enough Absorb Plus for the food reintroduction period. However, it's very difficult to calculate this ahead of time as the pace of food reintroduction will vary depending on how your body responds. Just try to estimate how much you'll need for this period and don't worry if you order too many as the shelf life for Absorb Plus (unopened) is about 2 years - so you'll have plenty of time to use up any extra stock. Also, some people like to drink one shake per day ongoing as a handy way to take their supplements and ensure ongoing good nutrition.

EXAMPLE:

Gillian wants to gain weight during the Diet and therefore needs to drink 6 Absorb Plus shakes per day for the first 3 weeks, then 7 Absorb Plus shakes per day for the next 3 weeks. She wants to stay on the diet for 6 weeks, which equals 42 days. Therefore, Gillian needs to order 28 tubs of Absorb Plus to last her the duration of the Diet (6 shakes x 21 days = 126 shakes and 7 shakes x 21 days = 147 shakes. So, 126 + 147 = 273 total shakes needed for 6 weeks. 273 shakes ÷ 10 = 27.3 tubs).

However, Gillian will also need to order enough Absorb Plus to see her through the food reintroduction phase. Depending on the pace of her food reintroduction, she'll need anywhere from 2 - 5 shakes per day, decreasing as she eats more and more solid food. Rather than trying to calculate this (as it's very hard to predict ahead of time), she's just going to order 5 extra tubs, so her total order will be 33 tubs of Absorb Plus.

Important: If she's short on cash, she can call the company and find out how long shipping takes and stagger her order, ordering 15 tubs or so at a time. But she'll need to be careful to make sure her second shipment arrives a few days before she actually needs it.

3

SUPPLEMENTATION PLAN & RECIPES

All things appear and disappear because of the concurrence of causes and conditions. Nothing ever exists entirely alone; everything is in relation to everything else.
Buddha

EACH OF THE RECOMMENDED supplements in the IBD Remission Diet has been chosen for its specific action on the immune and digestive system. The objective is twofold: 1) to rebuild the intestinal wall and mucosal lining and assist the healing of any wounds, ulcers, fissures, fistulas or diverticulae, and, 2) to support and balance the immune system so immune function returns to normal. Inflammatory Bowel Diseases (IBD) are all classed as auto-immune disorders; meaning that, for some unknown reason, the body attacks itself. This results in on-going wounding to the digestive tract which can include ulceration, fissures (deep cracks in the intestinal wall) and fistulas (cracks that penetrate right through the intestinal wall and can often join up with another crack that leads into a new section of intestine, or exit the gastrointestinal tract). Thus, part of healing IBD long-term involves healing and re-balancing the immune system so its function returns to its normal protective state. This is why I encourage you to wean off all prescription drugs prior to starting the IBD Remission Diet, so your body is able to reap the full benefits of the elemental diet, supplementation plan and probiotic flora replacement.

The other key facet of healing IBD (Inflammatory Bowel Disease) involves direct healing of any ulceration, fissures, fistulas and diverticulae by using herbs, vitamins, minerals, amino acids and other natural compounds that facilitate the healing of gastro-intestinal tissue and the mucosal lining. Diverticulae are pouches in the colon where food can get stuck and then infect/inflame the surrounding tissue. This condition is dramatically improved by increasing the muscle tone of the intestinal wall, rebuilding the mucosal lining and balancing the bacterial flora, all of which should occur by following the IBD Remission Diet.

As you've seen from the clinical trials presented in Chapter One, an elemental diet, on its own, results in disease remission and in some cases complete healing of the intestinal mucosal lining. The beauty of this program (when followed correctly and completely) is that you not only get the benefits of disease remission (provided by the elemental diet), but the comprehensive supplementation plan results in digestive and systemic healing as well. The two combined should keep you healthy and symptom-free for the foreseeable future - of course you also need to follow the Maintenance Diet and recommendations for ongoing health in Chapter Five.

HEALING IMPLANT ENEMA

If you're experiencing a lot of bleeding primarily from your colon, you may want to use this enema mixture as it's excellent for wound healing and works very quickly. Because it's an implant enema (rather than a cleansing enema), the goal is to keep the enema mixture inside your colon for as long as possible. Therefore, you'll have best results if you administer it first thing in the morning (after your morning bowel movement) or last thing at night, or whenever your bowel is likely to be the most clear of stool. You can buy disposable enema kits from any medical supply shop (or your naturopath/ doctor may have some in-house). These kits can actually be used more than once if you rinse thoroughly with hot water and clean the tip well.

The enema mixture consists of: 1 tsp. Comfrey powder, 1 tsp. Marshmallow Root powder and 1 tsp. Slippery Elm (inner bark) powder, mixed in ½ litre (2 cups) of filtered or spring water. An herb pharmacy should have all the ingredients, but they must be in powder form. The powders mix best if you put the whole mixture in a blender and whip it for 30 seconds. If you don't have a blender then just mix them as best you can in the water by squashing the lumps with a spoon. Heat the mixture on the stove until it reaches body temperature or, if you're whipping it in the blender, just use hot water. When the mixture is body temperature, or about the temperature of milk in a baby's bottle, pour it into the enema bag. You'll probably need someone to assist you in administering the enema, at least for the first few times.

Using the clamp on the enema tube stops the flow of liquid, as does holding the end of the tube higher than the bag. So let the mixture flow down almost to the end of the tube and then clamp it about a foot and a half from the end to shut off the flow. You want the mixture right at the end of the tube, so that when you insert it and release the flow into your colon you don't get a lot of air going in as well. You may find it easy to insert the tube into your anus, but I'm going to give you instructions that will make it as easy as possible for even the most sensitive of rectums.

Start by rinsing a washcloth in hot water, wring it out, then press it against your perianal area. The heat and moisture will cause the tissue to soften up. Next, use your fingers to apply Vitamin E oil (available in capsules, just puncture the end with a needle and squeeze out the oil) all round and inside your anus. Also apply it to the tip of the enema tube and about two inches along the length. You can use KY jelly instead, but I prefer the Vitamin E oil as it's also an excellent wound healer that will prevent or help to heal any anal/rectal fissures. Insert the enema tube gently into your rectum (about three inches should be sufficient) and then have your assistant slowly release the clamp, allowing the mixture to flow in at a comfortable rate. You may have to keep the flow quite slow for the first few times and stop it every now and again before you're able to continue. But as you get used to the enemas you'll be able to accept the liquid faster. When all the mixture has gone in, re-clamp the tube and withdraw the tip from your rectum.

Here are some tips that will really improve the ease and efficacy of the implant enema:

1. Lie down on your right side with one or two pillows (covered with a towel) under your bum/hips. Having your bum raised up enables you to use gravity to assist the flow of the enema mixture into your colon. Lying on your right side draws the liquid into the rest of your colon, reducing the pressure on your rectal canal.

2. Be sure to breathe deeply and relax your abdomen throughout (fear or apprehension causes us to tense up). Visualize the mixture flowing in around the whole length of your colon; imagine your colon welcoming it and helping it along.

3. After the mixture is inside your colon and you've withdrawn the enema tube, begin gently massaging the mixture around in your colon so it gets into all the folds and ridges of the intestinal wall. However, be sure to massage and stroke in a counter-clockwise direction; up the left side (descending colon), across the top (transverse colon) from left to right, and down the right side (ascending colon) towards the ileocecal valve and the small intestine. You massage in this direction because you don't want to cause a bowel movement, you want to prevent one, by massaging away from the rectum, not towards it.

4. The point of an implant enema is to hold the mixture inside your colon for as long as possible - ideally until all the liquid has been absorbed. Therefore, it's best if you can stay lying down with your bum raised on the pillows for as long as possible. You may also want to lie first on your right side for half an hour, then on your back for half an hour, then on your left side for half an hour, allowing the mixture to saturate the different parts of your colon.

The first time I tried this enema, I was able to hold it in for one hour, the next time, an hour and a half. By the fourth time, I could hold it till all the liquid was absorbed and then didn't have a bowel movement until three hours later. If you're bleeding from your colon, it's best if you can do this enema once (or even twice) a day. Once the bleeding stops, do it every second day for a week, then every third day for another week, then once a week for a month. If you find your anus/rectum getting sore from the tube then you may want to discontinue or administer it less. Again, it's your body; do what you feel is best.

I know there's been a fair amount of controversy in the popular media regarding Comfrey being harmful to the liver. With all due respect, this appears to me to be another example of a pharmaceutical/medical-backed hysteria over a product that's shown itself to be very safe over thousands of years of use. Why isn't the media trumpeting the 7,000 deaths in the U.S. from Aspirin every year and demanding its use be discontinued? Always look for the financial motivation.

I have consulted several respected naturopaths and herbalists and the consensus is that Comfrey taken internally in this manner is safe as long as it's not continued long-term. Therefore, don't use the Healing Implant Enema for longer than six months at a time. You can use it for six months, take a break of a month or two to allow your liver to cleanse and then you can resume usage. Obviously, it's highly unlikely that anyone is going to administer daily enemas for six months continuously anyway! However, if you still have reservations about using the Comfrey powder, you can replace it with 1 tsp. Plantain powder and 1 tsp. Calendula powder.

FISTULA HEALING

Some people develop fistulas in their rectal canal and these wounds penetrate right through the rectum and exit either into the vagina, or, outside the body around the tailbone area. The elemental diet provides fistulas with an ideal chance to heal naturally as the fecal matter is greatly reduced and mostly liquid. However, for a fistula in the rectal canal that exits outside the body, you can also provide additional herbal healing assistance for the wound. Here's a procedure you can follow to clear up a mildly infected rectal fistula and further speed healing of your fistula wound whilst on The IBD Remission Diet:

1. Bathe the area at least once a day in Epsom salts. Soak in warm/hot water up to your navel for at least 15 minutes. Make sure the wound is exposed to the water and you're not sitting on it during the bath. Use 1 cup of Epsom salts per bath and add 30 drops of Tea Tree essential oil to the running bath water.

Tea Tree oil (from the Australian Tea Tree) enhances skin function, is antifungal, antibiotic, antiviral, non-irritating and is useful for healing pus-filled wounds and many types of mild and chronic infection.

2. After soaking in the bath, use a soft washcloth to slough off any dead and purulent (pus-filled) skin, rinse the area again in the bath water, soak for another 5 minutes, and then gently pat dry.

3. Follow either a) or b) depending on whether your wound is infected or not:
   a) As long as the infection is present, cover the entire wounded area with Tea Tree salve and massage into the tissue as much as possible. Then leave the wound open to the air for as long as possible (sleep naked overnight). If you get leakage then sleep on a big towel or washable mattress pad, but make sure it's 100% cotton so the wound can breathe adequately.
   b) Once your infection is cleared up, massage Doctor Burt's Res-Q Ointment (also called Dr. Burt's Comfrey Salve available from Burt's Bees Inc. in health stores or at www.burtsbees.com) all over the wound and surrounding tissue. Rub in as much as possible. Then leave the wound open to the air for as long as possible (sleep naked overnight). If you get leakage then sleep on a big towel or washable mattress pad, but make sure it's 100% cotton so the wound can breathe adequately.

Comfrey is the most fantastic wound healer I've ever encountered. It heals so quickly that you need to make sure the infection is cleared before using, otherwise you run the risk of healing the infection inside the tissue – it heals that fast!

4. Get a supply of FissureHeal herbal suppositories from www.fissureheal.com (or see Appendix A for order details). Insert the suppository and push up far enough so the suppository is as close to the area of the fistula as possible. The suppositories contain effective wound healers like Slippery Elm, Marshmallow Root, Comfrey Root and Cocoa Butter. This will help to heal your fistula from the inside

while you sleep. I've used them myself on two separate occasions for rectal fissures and they work very well.

For maximum effectiveness, follow this 4-step regimen in the morning before you go to work and then last thing before bed. If that's too difficult, then just do it before bed - this is assuming you have the least number of bowel movements during the night, so maximum chance for undisturbed healing. If you have frequent bowel movements in the morning, then don't bother with the suppository, only use it at night, or whenever you have the least number of bowel movements - or the longest stretch between movements.

If your fistula exits into your vagina, you can douche before bed (or whenever your bowels are least active for the longest stretch of time) with a mixture of:

2 drops Tea Tree essential oil

1 cup warm water

If any irritation occurs, discontinue the Tea Tree oil and just douche with warm/hot water to cleanse the area. Follow this douche by inserting a FissureHeal suppository into your rectum and another into your vagina and positioning both in the area of your fistula. The suppositories contain Cocoa Butter which is a very rich emollient, so if you get vaginal itching due to too much moisturizer, then just insert the suppository into your rectum. Also, the Cocoa Butter can damage condoms so switch to another method of birth control if that's what you're using - or better yet, just abstain from intercourse to give your fistula the best chance for undisturbed healing.

WHICH SUPPLEMENTS & WHY?

The supplements you'll need to facilitate whole-body healing are listed below in point form and the amounts are given for each. Following these lists are detailed descriptions of each recommended supplement and how exactly they will benefit your immune system and digestive tract. I've given recommendations for good quality brands of each recommended supplement to make your shopping easier. However, please keep in mind that companies change their formulas, or can be bought up by less scrupulous companies and these formulas and standards of quality can change. So, at all times, double-check that the brand does indeed contain the form and amount of supplement recommended. As a general guideline, for children aged 2-6, administer ¼ of the recommended adult dose. For children aged 7-13, administer ½ the recommended adult dose. If you're unsure, consult your naturopathic physician. Consume these supplements for as long as you're drinking the shakes on the elemental diet. Even after you've completed the IBD Remission Diet, you may want to continue taking one shake a day with added supplements (see Recipe section for details) to maintain your health and support immune function.

Supplements to be Added to Absorb Plus Shakes:

- Alternate Coenzyme Q10 (30 mg. per shake) with Pycnogenol (30 mg. per shake) i.e. put CoQ10 in one shake, then Pycnogenol in the next and so on, to a combined maximum of 200 mg. per day.
- Vitamin C in mineral ascorbate (calcium ascorbate, magnesium ascorbate etc.) form (1000 mg. per shake to maximum of 10,000 mg. per day)
- Iron - if anemic (1 capsule/25 mg. 1-2 times per day, ferrous citrate is the best form of iron)
- Mixed Bioflavonoids containing approx. 50 mg. each of Rutin, Quercetin, Hesperidin (1 capsule per shake to a maximum of 6 capsules per day)

If you're not using Absorb Plus, you also need to add to each shake:
- Mixed Tocopherols Vitamin E, containing alpha, beta, delta, gamma tocopherols (total 400 IU per day)
- L-Glutamine (total approximately 6 grams per day - add 1 gram per shake)
- Vitamin B complex (total 30-50 grams per day)
- High quality multi-vitamin (1 capsule per shake)
- High quality multi-mineral (1 capsule per shake)

Between Shakes (on an empty stomach):

- George's Roadrunner Aloe Vera Juice (¼ cup 3 times/day while bleeding, otherwise, ¼ cup before bed)
- MucosaHeal - contains Licorice, Slippery Elm, Marshmallow Root, N-Acetyl Glucosamine (Follow dosage instructions on the bottle. Can be mixed with clear apple juice if you can't swallow pills). See Appendix A for order details.

Now that you know what you need to put in each shake (or take between shakes), let me explain why:

Coenzyme Q10

A powerful antioxidant, CoQ10 protects the heart and liver and is vital for many bodily functions. Since the liver is the main detoxification organ of the body, protecting and assisting the liver will also minimize damage to all body tissues. CoQ10 also aids circulation, increases tissue oxygenation and balances the immune system. It also counters histamine, so is beneficial for people with allergies or asthma. Japanese research has shown that CoQ10 protects the stomach lining and duodenum. Look for CoQ10 that is bright yellow to orange in color and keep it away from heat and light.

Pycnogenol

Pycnogenol is an oligomeric proanthocyanidin (OPC), produced from the French maritime pine tree. Grape seed extract is also an OPC and so can be used instead of Pycnogenol if you prefer (it's usually cheaper). OPCs are potent antioxidants that are able to cross the blood-brain barrier, therefore they can protect the brain and spinal nerves from free radical damage. They also protect the liver, strengthen and repair connective tissue and support the immune system. In addition, they reduce histamine production, benefitting those with allergies and other inflammatory responses.

Vitamin C

An antioxidant required for at least 300 different metabolic functions in the body, including adrenal gland function, tissue growth and repair, protection against infection, and cancer prevention. Literally hundreds of clinical studies (including double-blind and placebo controlled) have been done on Vitamin C to determine its safety and efficacy. It is one of the most beneficial substances you can take for your immune system. In one particularly memorable trial, researchers gave 60 patients with Polio intramuscular Vitamin C shots (1-2 grams every 2-4 hours, depending on the age of the patient, for the first 24 hours, then 1-2 grams every 6 hours for the next 48 hours) and within 72 hours every single one of them was diagnosed "clinically well". (*F. Klenner, "The Treatment of Poliomyelitis and Other Virus Diseases with Vitamin C", Journal of Southern Medicine and Surgery, Vol. 111, 1949, pp. 209-214*). If a drug could accomplish what Vitamin C does for our bodies, it would be all over the media, every doctor would prescribe it, and it would be part of nearly every hospital visit. Alas, as it's a natural, non-patentable substance, there's no exclusive, economic reward for promoting Vitamin C and, more importantly, its widespread use would cause billions of dollars in lost revenue for drugs and vaccines.

Vitamin C in its common ascorbic acid form causes diarrhea. Therefore, make sure you get a Vitamin C powder in mineral ascorbate form (e.g. calcium ascorbate, magnesium ascorbate, etc.). High doses of magnesium can also cause diarrhea, so get a higher proportion of calcium ascorbate if the two are mixed, or just get Vitamin C in calcium ascorbate form. The mineral ascorbate form is also preferable as it's more readily absorbed - ascorbic acid has to first be converted to mineral ascorbates by the body prior to absorption. Another delicious way to get your daily Vitamin C in mineral ascorbate form (for ongoing use) is by using Emergen-C (by Alacer Corp.) handy single-serving packets naturally flavored in your choice of tangerine, cranberry, raspberry, lemon-lime, etc. It is also compatible with an elemental diet. Emergen-C is a common product in any health store or see Appendix A for order details.

Iron

The absolute best iron supplement I have ever found is Ferrasorb by Thorne Research Inc. It is available only through your naturopath or naturopathic pharmacy and they make different formulas for Canada and the US. I've tried both and if you can, get the formula produced for Canada (containing Iron Citrate) as I find it a bit gentler on the stomach and very bland-tasting so it's easy to mix in your shakes without altering the taste. If you get the US formula (containing Iron Picolinate) then you may want to just swallow it on its own before drinking your shake. 3-4 capsules per day (25 mg. each) in divided doses (i.e. take one capsule in the morning, the other mid-afternoon, the third in the evening) should be sufficient to address even severe anemia. If you're mildly to moderately anemic, take 1-2 capsules per day (in divided doses if taking 2 or more per day).

Bioflavonoids

Bioflavonoids (including Rutin, Hesperidin and Quercetin) are plant compounds that act synergistically with Vitamin C to strength-en vein and capillary walls so they don't tear and bleed so easily. They are produced by plants to protect themselves from bacteria, parasites and cell injury. If your gums bleed when you brush your teeth, or your nose bleeds when it's dry or you blow it forcefully, or you're prone to anal or rectal fissures, then you definitely need to supplement with Bioflavonoids. Bioflavonoids have also been shown to reduce back and leg pain, promote circulation, treat and prevent cataracts, stimulate bile production, and lower cholesterol levels. Get a brand that contains about 50 mg. each of Rutin, Hesperidin and Quercetin. At this time, Eclectics Institute and Allergy Research Corp. both have good formulas. If you suffer from Hay Fever, take 400 mg. of Quercetin per day as Quercetin regulates histamine release from the cells and you'll see a big improvement (if not elim-ination) of your allergies.

Vitamin E

Vitamin E is a great tissue healer and can reduce scarring, it maintains healthy muscles and nerves and strengthens capillary walls. It also promotes healthy hair and skin and helps prevent anemia. It is also an antioxidant and thus far has been shown to protect against 80 different diseases. Low levels of Vitamin E have been linked to both bowel and breast cancer. Some studies have shown Vitamin E to be even more protective against heart attacks than aspirin.

L-Glutamine

The primary nutrient for cells that line the gastrointestinal tract, L-Glutamine is essential for DNA synthesis, cell division and cell growth, which are all necessary for wound healing and tissue repair. It readily crosses the blood-brain barrier so is also essential for proper brain activity and mental function. L-Glutamine helps to maintain the proper pH level in the body (acid/alkaline balance), enhances antioxidant protection and decreases sugar cravings and the desire for alcohol. The main function we're using it for here is to rebuild and repair the mucosal lining of the intestine. If you're using Absorb Plus, it automatically contains over 1 gram (1000 mg.) of pharmaceutical-grade L-Glutamine per serving. Otherwise, add 1 gram per shake.

Multi-Vitamins/Multi-Minerals

I could write a whole book on all the myriad beneficial and vital functions all the different vitamins and minerals perform in our bodies, but as the information is already widely available I'll leave it to you to do your own research if you want more details. The key reason I recommend high doses of vitamins and minerals during this diet is that most (if not all) people with IBD or IBS have vitamin and mineral deficiencies due to poor diet, lack of absorption, prescription drug use, etc. Some of you may even want to go beyond what I've recommended and investigate megadose, intravenous vitamin and mineral therapy (talk to your naturopath for more information on this), which has a long history of beneficial action in all kinds of disease states. Minerals also have an alkalizing effect on the body (reduce an acidic body pH level) and are therefore particularly good for people with Inflammatory Bowel Disease.

Once you're no longer consuming three or more Absorb Plus shakes per day, you'll need to supplement with a separate multi-vitamin/mineral. Nature's Way and Eclectics Institute have good formulas. Once you've supplemented regularly for one year, begin cycling your vitamin/mineral use with one month on and one month off. I recommend this because I believe the body's homeostatic mechanism will cause it to adjust to any substance taken long-term and the substance then won't be as effective. Therefore, if you cycle on and off and don't take anything continuously or long-term, you'll derive maximum benefit from those substances. However, if the majority of your food (especially fruits and vegetables) is not certified organic, then you may want to just take a multi-vitamin/mineral every day to ensure you're at least getting the minimum requirements.

Vitamins A and B-Complex

B-Complex vitamins are especially helpful for people with gastrointestinal problems as they are key players in the synthesis and repair of the mucosal lining and intestinal wall. B vitamins are also well-known for their ability to reduce muscle spasms, aid in red blood cell production, assist in the digestion and metabolism of fat, protein and carbohydrates and support the adrenal gland, thereby increasing the body's resistance to stress. Absorb Plus contains the entire B-Complex (including B12) in each serving, so if you're using Absorb Plus for your shakes you don't need to add additional B vitamins. Another key vitamin involved in the mucosal lining of the intestine is Vitamin A and Absorb Plus contains good levels of both Vitamin A and Beta Carotene per serving. Again, when you begin to taper off the diet and are consuming less than 3 Absorb Plus shakes per day, make sure you start supplementing with a multi-vitamin that has good levels of the A and B vitamins (at least 10-50 mg. of each B vitamin and 5,000 IU of Beta Carotene and 3,000 IU of

Vitamin A). If you're pregnant, don't consume more than 10,000 IU of Vitamin A per day.

George's Roadrunner Aloe Vera Juice

I have specified a particular brand of aloe vera juice here because none of the other aloe vera juice products I've seen match this formula. Other brands may claim to be superior to George's Roadrunner brand because they contain higher levels of certain active ingredients. However, these active ingredients, whilst beneficial in some ways, also cause diarrhea and other intestinal problems. So please, do NOT substitute another brand of aloe vera juice. George's Roadrunner works extremely well for people with IBD/IBS with no undesirable side effects. It is excellent for stopping intestinal bleeding and healing wounds and ulcers. Aloe vera also combats viral and bacterial infection. See Appendix A for order details for George's Roadrunner Aloe Vera Juice if it's not available in your local health store.

MucosaHeal

This is a fantastic product (available from www.mucosaheal.com) which needs to be taken on an empty stomach. As you can see from the description of ingredients below, it is wonderful for healing the gastro-intestinal tract and restoring the mucosal lining. Follow the instructions on the bottle as the dosage varies according to whether you're experiencing active bleeding and inflammation, or not.

Deglycyrrhizinated Licorice - reduces muscle spasms, promotes adrenal gland function, soothes inflammation and fights bacterial, viral and parasitic infection. Increases number of mucus-secreting cells in intestine which improves the quality of the mucosal lining, lengthens intestinal cell life and enhances micro-circulation in the gastrointestinal tract.

Slippery Elm - good for diarrhea and ulcers when taken internally. Soothes inflamed mucous membranes of the stomach, intestines and urinary tract.

Marshmallow Root - soothes and heals mucous membranes, skin and other tissues. Also aids the body in expelling excess mucus and fluid.

N-Acetyl Glucosamine (NAG) - an amino sugar that forms the basis of complex molecular structures that are key parts of the connective tissue and mucous membranes of the body - tendons, ligaments, cartilage, bone matrix, skin, synovial (joint) fluid, and intestinal lining. To maintain healthy absorption and digestion of food, the body needs a healthy mucosal lining to lubricate and protect the digestive tract. To keep this lining healthy the body uses the natural amino acids and sugars L-Glutamine and N-Acetyl Glucosamine. It is also an immune system modulator with anti-tumor properties.

Many of the supplements outlined above are automatically contained in Absorb Plus, therefore, for most of you, here's what your daily elemental shakes are going to be comprised of:

IBD Remission Diet Shake Recipe with Supplements

1. Pour one cup (8 oz) of cold or room-temperature spring or filtered water into a blender

2. Add 1 serving of Absorb Plus (100 grams/4 level scoops)

3. Add the supplements of your choice:
   - Alternate Coenzyme Q10 (30 mg. per shake) with Pycnogenol (30 mg. per shake) i.e. put CoQ10 in one shake, then Pycnogenol in the next and so on. To a combined maximum of 200 mg. per day.
   - Vitamin C in mineral ascorbate (calcium ascorbate, magnesium ascorbate etc.) form (1000 mg. per shake, to a maximum of 10,000 mg. per day)
   - Iron - if anemic (1 capsule/25 mg. 1-2 times per day, ferrous citrate is the best form of iron)
   - Mixed Bioflavonoids containing approx. 50 mg. each of Rutin, Quercetin, Hesperidin (1 capsule per shake to a maximum of 6 capsules per day)

4. Add 1 tsp. - 1 tbsp. of organic flax or Udo's oil (according to tolerance, to a maximum of 8 tablespoons per day)

5. Whip on high speed for 10-15 seconds

6. Pour into a glass over ice and drink through a straw (if you prefer).

Figure out how many shakes per day you need to consume to meet your nutritional and caloric needs (see Chapter Two) and together with the following broth and jello recipes, you're ready to begin the IBD Remission Diet. There are approximately ten servings/shakes in each 1 kg tub of Absorb Plus, so figure out how many shakes per day you're going to consume before you start the IBD Remission Diet and make sure you order enough Absorb Plus to see you through or at least cover you till the next delivery (the product is only available through direct mail order via a toll-free number or Internet). This is also a good idea because the company offers substantial bulk discounts if you buy three or more tubs at a time, so it will be much cheaper for you. Also, check with your health insurance company to see if they will provide partial or full coverage for the cost of the elemental shakes, as your doctor can give you a letter stating it's a medical necessity or his/her recommended course of treatment for your condition.

BROTH & JELLO RECIPES

Drink the following broths between shakes to provide added nutrients and taste variety. If you just consume sweet tastes all day (the shakes), your appetite won't be very stimulated and you may find it difficult to drink the number of shakes you need each day, or to stick with the diet for any length of time. Alternating with a 'salty' taste stimulates the appetite and makes you ready for the next sweet shake. A bowl of broth contains minimal calories so you can eat as many as you like. The taste of these broths is superb and you'll probably find yourself continuing to use them even after you finish the diet. However, if you don't want to make broths from scratch, you can buy them in cans or cartons. Just make sure the broths are clear, all-natural, and certified organic.

The dieticians I've talked to maintain that broths are pretty much empty calories. However, my intuitive feeling (and feedback from readers) is that broths made from scratch are very nutritious and healing. While I've never read anything scientific on the benefits of consuming bone marrow or gelatin, my intuition and body tells me they're very sustaining and constitutional, and they are traditionally revered. I once received a letter from a reader telling me how the Beef Broth "saved her life" when she was recovering from severe haemorrhaging and malnutrition.

The Mushroom Broth reminds me of the Chinese practice of boiling herbs or mushrooms to make medicinal teas. The cell walls of mushrooms contain polysaccharides in a form called beta-glucans. Beta-glucans are released from the chitin (polysaccharide that forms the skeleton of mushrooms) by cooking and the best way is to boil them into a broth. Beta-glucans have antitumor, antiviral, antibacterial, antifungal and antiparasitic actions. However, you need to eat the mushrooms while they're fresh, so either consume within a week of purchase, or use dried mushrooms (drying preserves the nutrients).

So, although it's a bit of work, I do encourage you to make these broths from scratch rather than buying pre-packaged versions.

If you're very weak, get a family member or friend to make some up for you - don't hesitate to ask for help! I also strongly recommend you use only certified organic meat and produce for these broths, if at all possible. Since you're boiling down and concentrating all the meat, skin and bones, it's best if you use healthy, non-toxic ingredients - especially since your own body is so vulnerable at this time. Also, try to get the finest mesh strainer you can as this will help remove all the little bits from your broth, leaving it as clear as possible.

Chicken Broth

1. Rinse one whole certified organic chicken inside and out with cold water and remove any giblets or organs that have been placed inside the rib cavity (do not use these, although you can throw the neck into the pan with the chicken if that's included). Place chicken in roasting pan and sprinkle 1 tsp. of basil and 1 tsp. oregano on top. Add 1 cup of spring or filtered water (no tap water). Preheat oven to 350 degrees, cover pan and cook for one and a half hours.

2. Take the pan out of the oven and cut away as much of the meat as you wish. Refrigerate and use the meat for meals for the rest of your family and/or divide into desired portion sizes and freeze in zip-lock plastic bags for later use (allow chicken to cool down before sealing in plastic bags).

3. Cut and mash up the remaining chicken parts, skin and bones in the pan, add 6 more cups of spring or filtered water, 1 tsp. sea salt, and mix well. Cover and cook at 350 degrees for another 45 minutes.

4. Remove pan from oven, mix well and then pour contents through a fine strainer into a large bowl (throw out chicken remnants). Place this large bowl uncovered in the fridge for about 12 hours, or until broth has become jelly-like and the fat has risen and solidified, or thickened, on top.

5. Skim fat off top of bowl with a spoon (throw away fat). Portion up the remaining chicken soup jelly into individual servings in zip-lock plastic bags and put them in the freezer to use as needed. Don't worry about making too much because even when you're back on regular food, this chicken broth is excellent as a stock for soups, sauces, etc. If, for some reason, you absolutely cannot use a certified organic chicken for this broth, then follow the same procedure for a non-organic chicken but DO NOT boil the bones or skin, as directed in point 3. The bones and skin of a non-organic chicken are too toxic, so just pull off all the meat and boil that.

Stovetop Chicken Broth

If you don't have a roasting pan, you can make the chicken broth in a large pot with a lid on the stovetop instead. The taste won't be as nice though as you don't get the roasted flavor.

1. Rinse one whole certified organic chicken inside and out with cold water and remove any giblets or organs that have been placed inside the rib cavity (do not use these, although you can throw the neck into the pot with the chicken if that's included). Add spring or filtered water (no tap water) to a depth of one inch, around the chicken (i.e. you should have one inch of water in the bottom of the pot). Sprinkle top of chicken with a bit of garlic powder and salt. Cover pot with the lid, bring to a boil on high heat, then reduce heat and gently simmer covered (low, gentle boil) for one and a half to two hours. This results in a 'pot roast' effect for the chicken. You can tell when the chicken is fully cooked by pulling on a leg - if the leg tears away easily, then it is well done. It is not necessary to add any more water to the pot while you're cooking the chicken, as the water level will remain the same, or increase as juices are released from the chicken.

2. Remove the pot from heat and cut away as much of the meat as you wish. Refrigerate and use the meat for meals for the rest of your family and/or divide into desired portion sizes and freeze in zip-lock plastic bags for later use (allow chicken to cool down before sealing in plastic bags).

3. Put all the remaining chicken parts, skin and bones back in the pot with its juices, add 4 more cups of spring or filtered water, 1 tsp. sea salt, and mix well. Replace the lid and simmer gently for another 30 minutes

4. Remove pot from heat, mix well and then pour contents through a fine strainer into a large bowl (throw out chicken remnants). Place this large bowl uncovered in the fridge for about 24 hours, or until broth has become jelly-like and the fat has risen and solidified, or thickened, on top. Or, place in the freezer for only 6 hours to make removal of the fat from the top very easy.

5. Skim fat off top of bowl with a spoon (throw away fat). Portion up the remaining chicken soup jelly into individual servings in zip-lock plastic bags and put them in the freezer to use as needed. Don't worry about making too much because even when you're back on regular food, this chicken broth is excellent as a stock for soups, sauces, etc. If, for some reason, you absolutely cannot use a certified organic chicken for this broth, then follow the same procedure for a non-organic chicken but DO NOT use a whole chicken. The bones and skin of a non-organic chicken are too toxic, so when you get to step 3, just put chicken meat only in the pot and simmer that as directed above.

Vegetable Broth

1. Wash and chop up a saucepan-full of certified organic carrots, zucchini, and broccoli (including stalks). You can also add any other certified organic vegetables you like. Add spring or filtered water (no tap water) to one inch over the top of vegetables and 1 tsp. salt. Cover, bring to a boil, then turn down the heat and simmer for 1 hour. Remove from heat and pour through a fine strainer into a large bowl.

2. Allow broth to cool then divide up the liquid into individual servings and freeze in zip-lock plastic bags. Tastes really good on its own or mixed with Chicken or Beef Broth. When you're back eating regular food it's also a great stock for soups or sauces.

3. The remaining vegetables can be used, if you wish, (although the nutrient level will be really low) for meals for the rest of your family. For example: Spread them out in a pan and grate Cheddar and Monterey Jack cheese over the top, broil until cheese is melted and serve.

Beef Broth

1. Take a piece of certified organic beef (get the bloodiest, lowest-fat cut you can afford) and put it in a pot. Add water till it covers the meat, add 1 tsp. basil, 1 tsp. oregano. Cover and simmer this on the stovetop at a low boil.

2. Simmer for two hours, adding water as needed to keep the meat covered at all times. Then add 1 tsp. salt and simmer covered for 30 minutes.

3. Remove from heat and pour the contents of the pot into a fine strainer, catching the broth in another pot or bowl underneath. Add additional salt to taste. If your broth has visible fat in it, skim the fat off first before eating, or put the soup in the fridge until the fat solidifies on the top, and then you can just lift it off easily.

4. Allow broth to cool then divide up into individual servings and freeze in zip-lock plastic bags. Tastes really good on its own or mixed with vegetable broth. When you're back eating regular food it's also a great stock for soups, stews or sauces.

Steak Broth

The best tasting steak broth is obtained by using certified organic Sirloin Steak, but any certified organic cut can be used.

- Approximately 9 ounces (.3 kg) organic Sirloin Steak
- 1 tbsp. organic butter
- sprinkle of garlic powder
- sprinkle of salt
- 4 cups spring or filtered water
- 1 tsp. salt

1. Sprinkle a light dusting of salt and garlic powder on one side of the steak

2. Bring 1 tbsp. butter to bubbling in a pan on medium high heat, then place steak in the pan, seasoned side down.

3. Sprinkle the top of the steak with a light dusting of salt and garlic powder and when the underside is browned, flip the steak over and brown the other side. When browned, remove from heat.

4. Place steak on a plate and slice into thin slices (including fat and gristle), retaining all the blood and juices that are released.

5. Return everything to the frying pan and add 4 cups water and 1 tsp. salt. Cover and simmer for ½ hour.

6. Remove from heat, then pour through a fine strainer to catch the broth in a bowl underneath. Add salt to taste. Either consume immediately or refrigerate or freeze broth for future use.

7. To reuse the steak, marinate the slices in 1 tbsp. soy sauce and use in a stir-fry, or, just add salt and pepper and use in sandwiches.

Mushroom Broth
(fabulous as a tonic for the immune system)

Try to get a mix of certified organic mushrooms as mushrooms tend to concentrate heavy metals (including lead) if these substances are present in the growth medium. But if none are available, then non-organic mushrooms are okay. You can also use dried mushrooms instead of fresh if you prefer - follow instructions on the label for rehydrating and then use the same water to boil the mushrooms in. Reishi and Maitake mushrooms are also fantastic sources of beta-glucans so if you can find them definitely include them in your broth. Button mushrooms don't really have any health benefits, but I've included them for flavor as they're much cheaper than the other mushrooms.

- 2 cups each of Shiitake, Oyster, Portobello, and Button mushrooms (sliced and pressed down in the measurement cup)
- 3 tablespoons organic butter
- ¼ tsp. garlic powder
- 1 and ½ tsp. sea salt
- 8 cups of filtered or spring water

1. Melt the butter in a large frying pan, add the mushrooms, garlic powder and ½ tsp. of salt. Fry on medium high heat, stirring frequently, until mushrooms are just beginning to brown.

2. Add all 8 cups of water and 1 tsp. of salt, cover and boil the mixture gently for 30 minutes, stirring once or twice.

3. Strain broth by pouring contents of pan into a bowl through a fine sieve. Either portion up and freeze in zip-lock plastic bags (allow broth to cool first before pouring into plastic), or store in a glass jar in the fridge. Mushroom broth will stay fresh, refrigerated, for up to one week. You can add additional salt if you wish.

4. To reuse the mushrooms for the rest of the family, drain and cool them and then cut off the stems of the Shiitake and Oyster mushrooms (these are too tough to eat). Return them to the pan and

fry for about 2 minutes with 1 tsp. butter, 1/4 tsp. salt and a little garlic. The mushrooms can then be eaten as is, or used in a pasta sauce, stir-fry or casserole, etc.

Natural Jello

1. Pour one pouch of Knox unflavored gelatin (1 tbsp. gelatin) over 1/4 cup of natural, unsweetened, clear, fruit juice (preferably certified organic).

2. Add 1/4 cup boiling water and stir constantly until gelatin is completely dissolved (about 1-2 minutes).

3. Add another 1.5 cups of juice, stir and refrigerate until set.

   ★ *If you want a stiffer jelly, then add less juice*

Shake Recipes

These shake recipes will give you a bit of flavor variety while you're on the elemental diet. Always use level scoops when measuring Absorb Plus, and don't forget to add your supplements as well:

Choco-Berry Shake

1. Pour 1 cup (8 ounces) of cold water into a blender

2. Add:

    - 2 scoops Absorb Plus Chocolate Royale flavor
    - 2 scoops Absorb Plus Mixed Berry flavor
    - any supplements you wish to add
    - 1 tsp. - 1 tbsp. organic flax oil (as much as you can tolerate)

3. Whip on high speed for 10-15 seconds

4. Pour into a glass over ice and drink slowly.

Choco-Berry Shake for
People with a Chocolate Sensitivity

If chocolate tends to be hard on your system, but yet you still really love it, this reduced-chocolate shake recipe may work for you.

1. Pour 1 cup (8 ounces) of cold water into a blender

2. Add:

   • 1 scoop Absorb Plus Chocolate Royale flavor
   • 3 scoops Absorb Plus Mixed Berry flavor
   • any supplements you wish to add
   • 1 tsp. - 1 tbsp. organic flax oil (as much as you can tolerate)

3. Whip on high speed for 10-15 seconds

4. Pour into a glass over ice and drink slowly.

Chocolate Shake for
People with a Chocolate Sensitivity

If chocolate tends to be hard on your system, but yet you still really love it, here's another reduced-chocolate shake recipe that may work for you.

1. Pour 1 cup (8 ounces) of cold water into a blender

2. Add:

   - 1 scoop Absorb Plus Chocolate Royale flavor
   - 3 scoops Absorb Plus French Vanilla flavor
   - any supplements you wish to add
   - 1 tsp. - 1 tbsp. organic flax oil (as much as you can tolerate)

3. Whip on high speed for 10-15 seconds

4. Pour into a glass over ice and drink slowly.

ADDITIONAL DAILY SHAKE RECIPES

The following shake recipes are for you to use after you've finished the elemental diet and are eating regular food. For added health and nutritional support, I suggest you continue to take one shake per day, three a week, or just whenever you feel you need it:

Immune Support Shake

For vitamins in capsule form, open or puncture capsule and empty contents into shake, discard empty capsule shell.

1. Pour 1 cup (8 ounces) of cold water into a blender

2. Add:
    *   4 scoops Absorb Plus French Vanilla or Mixed Berry flavor
    *   1 capsule of mixed 50 mg. B-complex vitamins (B vitamins are quite strong-tasting, so you may wish to swallow this capsule separately)
    *   1000 mg. Vitamin C powder in Mineral Ascorbate form only (e.g. preferably as Calcium Ascorbate)
    *   400 IU capsule of mixed tocopherols Vitamin E (alpha, beta, delta, gamma tocopherols)
    *   1 capsule of CoQ10 or Pycnogenol, 60 mg.
    *   1 tsp. - 1 tbsp. Udo's Choice Perfected Oil Blend (as much as you can tolerate)

3. Whip on high speed for 10-15 seconds

4. Pour into a glass over ice and drink slowly.

Custom-Make Your Shake

Here is another shake for you to use once you've finished the elemental diet and are eating normal food again. You may still wish to take one shake a day (or 3 times per week) for added nutritional and health support. Perhaps you have some other health concerns that require specific supplements and this is a great, easily absorbed way to take them. For vitamins in capsule form, open or puncture capsule and empty contents into shake, discard empty capsule shell. Do not add 'greens' products (spirulina, algae, wheatgrass, etc) to this shake as it will ruin the taste.

1. Pour 1 cup (8 ounces) of cold water (or milk substitute if you prefer) into a blender

2. Add:
    *   4 scoops Absorb Plus French Vanilla or Mixed Berry flavor
    *   1-2 capsules of your regular multi-vitamin/multi-mineral
    *   Any other supplements you want to add (eg. anti-oxidants, ginko, ginseng, etc.)
    *   1 tsp. - 1 tbsp. Udo's Choice Perfected Oil Blend or organic flax oil (as much as you can tolerate)

3. Whip on high speed for 10-15 seconds

4. Pour into a glass over ice and drink slowly.

TAKE ACTION

Make a list here of the different supplements you need to purchase before beginning the IBD Remission Diet. You need to include supplements that go in the shakes, supplements that you take between shakes, and suppositories (if you need them to heal fissures or fistulas):

_____

_____

_____

_____

_____

_____

_____

_____

_____

_____

_____

_____

Make your grocery list here for the broths and jello you want to make. Depending on how long you're going to be on the Diet, you may want to make up numerous batches of each broth in advance, as it's easier to just make more, all at once, than one batch at a time. Also, do you have all the pots and pans you'll need? Don't forget to put freezer-safe Ziplock bags on your list if you don't have them to hand (or you can use glass jars to freeze the broths in):

_____

_____

_____

_____

_____

_____

_____

_____

_____

_____

_____

4

FOOD REINTRODUCTION & ALLERGY TESTING

We tend to see our own experiences as the normal process, so we are often amazed that anyone could have taken a different path. But when we do meet up, it's always fascinating to compare notes about the different ways to get there.
Daniel Gilly

Once you've been on the strictly elemental diet for the required period of time (see Chapter Two), you can then begin to introduce solid foods to your diet again. This is a good time to thoroughly test for possible allergic reactions or food intolerances. If you're not concerned about that, then you can introduce foods faster, or in groups, rather than one at a time. However, as most people with IBD/IBS have food intolerances, I'm going to give detailed instructions on food reintroduction and allergy/intolerance testing in this section.

UNDESIRABLE REACTIONS

After you've cleared most or all of your symptoms on the elemental diet, you can then reintroduce regular foods, one food at a time, and check for any abnormal reactions. Reacting in these ways to consuming a food shows that your body has either an allergy or intolerance to that food. These reactions can lessen or even disappear as your health improves over time, but it's good to keep them in mind as during times of stress they'll likely resurface and you'll want to avoid or minimize these foods again. Undesirable reactions to watch for include:

- increased mucus production
- nausea, itchy tongue or skin, swelling, redness, bumps, rash
- bloating/gas, cramps
- heartburn, indigestion
- shortness of breath, fuzzy head or a drugged feeling, sleepiness, etc.
- headache, joint/muscle pain
- any blood mixed in with or accompanying stool. Blood from the colon or rectum will be red. Blood from the small intestine will turn the stool dark green or black (as can iron therapy/supplements, so don't confuse the two). If you only have a bit of blood on the toilet paper when you wipe your bum, it's probably from a minor anal or rectal fissure/wound so don't worry about it.

Once you've been eating completely solid food for a minimum of two weeks, you can also check for these undesirable reactions:

- undigested particles of the test food in the stool or toilet bowl
- watery, slimy, or acidic stool
- increased diarrhea

It doesn't make any sense to monitor for these reactions while you're still consuming the elemental shakes, as the liquid shakes themselves can cause these same reactions for the following reasons: Firstly, consuming elemental shakes results in liquid fecal matter and liquid fecal matter results in more urgent, liquid bowel movements (diarrhea). The urgency of the liquid bowel movement also speeds the transit time of the stool through the colon, leaving less time for the water to be re-absorbed and less time for digestion to take place - resulting in more undigested particles and watery stool. Also, it's good to keep in mind that people with completely normal bowel function have undigested food particles in their stool too. If stool is formed and solid, the food particles are not noticeable, but they're still there. My husband has a completely healthy digestive system and he will sometimes see bits of vegetables, corn, salad, etc. in certain bowel movements (but only because I've asked him to look, he never noticed these things before). My son also has very healthy bowels and when he poops in the toilet I can't see anything in his stool. However, when he poops in his diaper and the stool gets all mushed up, I can see all kinds of undigested food particles; flax seeds, mushrooms that he hasn't chewed up, red pepper skin, etc. Which reminds me; remember that digestion begins with enzymes in your saliva, so be sure to chew your food really well - ideally don't swallow the mouthful until the whole bolus is smooth mush. Chewing your food really well will also reduce the amount of undigested food particles in your stool.

The following Food Reintroduction Chart gives you a detailed plan of the order in which to introduce and test foods/beverages. The foods are divided up into four progressive phases and each phase has progressive subcategories of foods from A to E. Therefore, you would start with a food from category A in Phase 1. After you've tested all the foods in category A, you would move on to category B in Phase 1, and so on. When you get to the end of all the foods in Phase 1, it's a good idea to stay with just those foods for one to three weeks to allow your body to stabilize and establish a good foundation. Next, you start introducing the foods in Phase 2, and again, you start with a food from category A. Continue on in this manner until you get to the end of Phase 4. There are spices, oils and sweeteners listed throughout the different phases. If you feel a substance would be okay for you to try earlier, then go ahead. Please refer to pages 100-101 for the Food Reintroduction Chart.

When reintroducing foods after being solely on the IBD Remission Diet, you start with the most easily tolerated foods first, in their most easily digestible form. For example, the first food you try from Phase 1, category A may be carrots. So you would cook them well (don't try vegetables raw until the end of Phase 4) and then mash or puree them to begin with, or just chew each mouthful really, really well. You may eat only carrots once or twice a day, while continuing with the elemental diet, for 2-3 days before classifying carrots as "safe". Or you may choose to trial test a different food each day, until you're up to seven foods and then eat only those seven foods for another week to be sure. There are many ways and combinations of introducing and testing foods, use your intuition to determine the right pace of food reintroduction for you. Just remember to keep taking the elemental diet shakes (with all the supplements added) until you're on enough solid food to make up your required daily calorie count. It's extremely helpful during this time to keep a food journal of exactly what you eat, time of day, the way you feel physically, the way you feel emotionally, number and type of bowel movements, any undesirable reactions, etc.

You'll notice that wheat, dairy, potatoes and corn are not introduced until Phase 3 and 4. This is because they are the most common food allergens for people with IBD/IBS. In a clinical trial, thirty-three Crohn's patients were first put on TPN (Total Parenteral Nutrition - liquid nutrients given intravenously) to clear their symptoms. The researchers then gradually reintroduced one food per day to determine which foods were tolerated and which triggered a return of symptoms. Wheat was the highest offender (69%), then dairy products (48%), followed by yeast (31%), corn (24%) and potato (17%). (*Workman EM, Jones AJ, Hunter JG. Diet in the Management of Crohn's Disease. Human Nutr. 1984:38A:469-473*) If you suspect an allergy to one or more of these foods, you may want to test them at the very end, after you've been on Phase 1-4 foods for a month or two. However, if you've adjusted your diet to get along happily without them, then you may not want to start eating them again. Alternatively, if you feel dairy, wheat or potatoes would not be a problem for you, then feel free to test them earlier. Dairy products made from cow's milk are particularly allergenic for many people; goat's milk or cheese, or rice milk, are usually better tolerated. Also keep in mind that about 60% of the people who are allergic to dairy are also allergic to soy. I find I can tolerate and digest raw cow's milk (or cheese made from raw milk) very easily, but I have a very limited tolerance for pasteurized cow's milk. This is probably because the pasteurization process destroys the natural enzymes and bacteria in the cow's milk that facilitate digestion.

If you've been on the IBD Remission Diet mainly for the purpose of wound healing, or disease remission and you're not so concerned about testing for food allergies, then you can be a lot less structured when it comes to eating solids again. However, you may still want to use the Food Reintroduction Chart as a general guideline. Follow the same process as outlined above, testing different foods and waiting for a reaction and gradually increasing your solid intake as you gradually decrease the number of shakes per day. Alternatively, for a completely unstructured but relatively 'safe' reintroduction to food you could use the Reduce Diarrhea Diet from my *LISTEN TO YOUR GUT* book - just eat the foods/beverages as advised there. Once you've introduced all those foods, then follow the Minimize Gas & Bloating Diet (also from *LISTEN TO YOUR GUT*) and then lastly, follow the Maintenance Diet outlined in Chapter Five following.

It's quite an undertaking to follow an elemental diet and then go through the time-consuming, systematic reintroduction of food. However, nothing will help you get to the foundation of your unique body and what works for you better than this. Some people can completely clear all their symptoms using the IBD Remission Diet, and then the food testing process will hopefully help them stay that way. Some people can achieve remission on the IBD Remission Diet, but to permanently clear their condition involves further healing using herbal supplements and other therapies presented in *LISTEN TO YOUR GUT* (www.caramal.com), along with some necessary emotional healing.

It's very helpful to keep a Food Diary. Write down exactly what you eat and drink, when, how much, and how you felt at the time. At the end of the day, critique what you ate and how you feel. Describe the type, consistency, and number of bowel movements. Write down any other observations regarding gas, pain, bloating, bleeding, cramping, etc. Also, very important is to note your emotional state and any disturbing or stressful situations, thoughts, or feelings that occurred. Remember that mind/body/spirit are one, and food is not the only factor that influences your digestive system. You may want to buy a notebook and set it up something like this, or else just make photocopies of the Food Journal (on pages 98-99), and staple together to form a booklet.

Food allergies and intolerances are not just a physical phenomenon. People with multiple personalities can go into anaphylactic shock if they consume a certain food while in one personality. But in another personality, they can eat as much of that food as they want with no adverse effect. Or, someone can develop an allergy in direct response to a traumatic event. I once read about a woman who was eating grapes at the time she was told her mother had just died in a car accident. From that moment on, she could no longer eat grapes without experiencing a severe allergic reaction.

With food intolerances, some foods are okay if you eat them once a week, for example. But if you eat them three times a week you'll experience an adverse reaction. This is why individual testing is so important. I consulted an MD who specialized in food allergy testing and had written a book on holistic treatment methods, and he gave me his opinion on the following allergy testing methods. Blood allergy tests - which test for an immune response of IgE and IgG antibodies when the blood is exposed to the test food - have an accuracy rate of approximately 60-65%, in his experience. Skin allergy testing - where a minute amount of the food is inserted under the skin and then assessed for any reaction - has an accuracy rate of about 80%. The systematic reintroduction and testing of foods outlined here is the most reliable, accurate method.

However, keep in mind that some reactions can take up to three days to manifest after having eaten the test food. So your pace of reintroduction depends on how thorough you want your testing to be. Also, as your health gradually improves over time by using natural healing methods that support whole-body health, you'll find yourself no longer allergic or intolerant to the same number of foods. As your overall health improves, you'll be able to consume a larger variety of previously 'forbidden' foods.

Whichever method of food reintroduction you choose; whether it's a slow, methodical, testing for allergy method, or a quicker, less structured method, you MUST begin supplementing with probiotics (good bacteria) as soon as you begin eating solid foods again. See the following chapter for full details.

FOOD JOURNAL

Day: _____

Food Ingested: _____

Time:_____

Reactions:

    ☐ Increased mucus production

    ☐ Nausea

    ☐ Itchy tongue or skin, swelling, redness

    ☐ Bloating/gas, cramps

    ☐ Diarrhea (and number of movements:_____)

    ☐ Heartburn, indigestion

    ☐ Shortness of breath

    ☐ Fuzzy head or drugged feeling, sleepiness

    ☐ Headache, joint/muscle pain

    ☐ Undigested particles of test food in stool or toilet bowl

    ☐ Slimy, mucousy, or acidic stool

    ☐ Blood in stool or toilet (describe: _____

_____)

Number and type of bowel movements: _____

Emotional events or feelings:

_____

_____

_____

_____

_____

_____

_____

Anything else:

_____

_____

_____

_____

_____

_____

FOOD REINTRODUCTION CHART

Phase One				
A	B	C	D	E
Carrots	White rice	Sole	Pears	Vitamins
Squash	Rice noodles	Cod	Canteloupe	Minerals
Zucchini	Rice flour	Halibut	Apples	Basil
Mushrooms	Rice cakes	Sea bass	Olive oil	Thyme
Cucumber	Rice cereal	Monkfish	Flax oil	Oregano
	Rice milk	Tuna	Safflower oil	Salt
		Salmon	Hemp oil	Stevia
		Turkey	Sunflower oil	Fructose
		Trout		Turbinado sugar
		Chicken		Maple syrup

Phase Two				
A	B	C	D	E
Peas	Rice pancakes	Plums	Dill	Tapioca
Snow peas	Sweet rice	Watermelon	Sesame oil	Baking powder
Asparagus	Jasmine rice	Mangoes	Soy sauce	Baking soda
Green beans	Millet	Papaya	Eggs	Arrowroot flour
Yellow beans	Amaranth	Banana	Rosemary	
Amaranth	Buckwheat	Peaches	Garlic	
Bean sprouts	Quinoa	Avocado	Cilantro	
Yams	Spelt	Honeydew		
Sweet potato	Brown rice			
Pumpkin	Basmati rice			
Water chestnuts	Rice bread			

Phase Three

A	B	C	D	E
Butter lettuce	Soy milk	Peanuts	Mint	Daikon
Cauliflower	Soybeans	Cashews	Ginger	Bay leaf
Broccoli	Tofu	Walnuts	Paprika	Mustard
Celery	Soy flour	Raisins	Turmeric	Olives
Chives	Kamut	Blueberries	Lemon, Limes	Yoghurt
Spinach	Beef	Cranberries	Vanilla	Kefir
Bok choy	Pork	Apricots	Cinnamon	Goat milk
Seaweed, Nori	Lamb	Cherries	Saffron	Leeks
Bamboo shoots	Miso	Almonds	Coconut	Butter
	Duck	Nectarines		Goat cheese
	Goose	Strawberries		
	Sardines			
	Anchovies			

Phase Four

A	B	C	D	E
Artichokes	Beans	Wheat	Grapes	Cornstarch
Turnip	Lentils	Cous-cous	Pineapple	Vinegar
Parsnip	Beets	Plantain	Prunes	Lotusroot
Potatoes	Cabbage	Currants	Shrimp	Wasabi
Tomatoes	Chard, Kale	Figs, Dates	Prawns	Pickles
Lettuce	Kohlrabi	Oranges	Scallops	Ketchup
Onions	Rhubarb	Grapefruit	Lobster	Cumin
Brussel sprouts	Corn	Raspberries		Cheese
		Blackberries		Cow's milk

TAKE ACTION

☐ Photocopy the Food Journal pages and staple together to form a book (or get Kinko's to spiral bind it for about $3), or, start your own food journal in your own notebook.

List here any foods/drinks you already know you have an intolerance to. Make sure you don't introduce these foods until Phase 4 of the Food Reintroduction Chart:

_____

_____

_____

_____

_____

_____

_____

_____

_____

_____

_____

In the past, which 'Undesirable Reactions' have you experienced as a result of eating foods/drinks you're intolerant or allergic to?

_____

_____

_____

_____

_____

_____

_____

_____

_____

_____

Using the Food Reintroduction Chart, which 3 foods are you going to introduce/test first?

_____

_____

_____

5

PROBIOTICS & LONG-TERM HEALTH

*T*o array a man's will against
his sickness is the supreme art of medicine.
Henry Ward Beecher

A S I DESCRIBED IN in Chapter Two, one of the principle theories behind the deterioration of intestinal health is an imbalance of gut bacteria which leads to Leaky Gut Syndrome. If you get too much 'bad' bacteria in your gut and not enough 'good' bacteria, the bad bacteria will degrade the mucosal lining and even penetrate through the intestinal wall. This causes undigested particles of food to pass directly into the bloodstream where they are perceived as allergens and trigger an immune response. Good bacteria, on the other hand, promote intestinal health by forming a protective coating of the mucosal cell lining. Damaging substances like unhealthy bacteria, toxins, chemicals and wastes are filtered out and eliminated. Simultaneously, water and nutrients are absorbed (once properly digested) into circulation and made available to the billions of cells in the body that need them. A healthy gut flora also helps prevent yeast, fungus or parasites from adhering to the intestinal wall and causing problems.

Long-term intestinal/digestive health is impossible without a healthy bacterial flora in your small and large intestine. This is why it's crucial to supplement with probiotics (good bacteria) after you've been on the elemental diet, or after a course of antibiotic medication. The elemental diet starves off most of the bacteria in your gut since virtually no food passes into the colon for the bacteria to eat. Therefore, the IBD Remission Diet provides an excellent clearing of most of the bad/unhealthy bacteria in your gut that have been causing/contributing to your IBD/IBS. The supplements you consume whilst on the elemental diet rebuild and restore your intestinal wall and mucosal cell lining. If you follow this healing of your digestive tract with probiotic supplementation (and a healthy diet and lifestyle) you will ensure the health and integrity of your gut is maintained in the long term.

WHEN DO I START PROBIOTIC SUPPLEMENTATION?

All bacteria feed off the food that passes through the small and large intestine. Therefore, there's no point in supplementing with probiotics until you start eating solid food again. However, as soon as you come off the exclusively elemental diet and take your first bite of regular food, you need to start supplementing with probiotics. Continue supplementation through the gradual transition to completely solid food and then keep supplementing for an additional two months once you're completely on regular food. Thereafter, you will probably only need to supplement with probiotics once or twice a week to maintain your healthy gut flora, or maybe only once or twice a month - let your bowel movements and intestinal health be your guide. If your stools are well-formed and sit on the bottom of the toilet and you only have one to three bowel movements per day, then your bacterial flora is healthy and balanced and you don't need additional probiotic supplementation. You should also have little to no flatulence, but if you are experiencing gas or bloating, then supplement with probiotics. If you regularly eat organic yoghurt containing healthy bacteria, then you may not need to supplement with additional probiotics at all after the two month period, as the yoghurt alone may keep your intestines supplied with enough ongoing healthy bacteria.

WHICH PROBIOTICS DO I TAKE AND HOW OFTEN?

It's important to supplement with a full-spectrum probiotic that contains strains for both the small and large intestine. At the least, you need to take acidophilus and bifidum bacteria. My favorite probiotic manufacturer is Natren. If you can swallow pills, take their Trenev capsules as they contain an excellent full spectrum of probiotics and that's all you need to take. For children, or if you can't swallow pills, or if you suffer from heartburn, buy the Bifido Factor

(B. bifidum bacteria) and Mega Dophilus (L. acidophilus bacteria) and Digesta Lac (L. bulgaricus bacteria) powders and mix them together in filtered room-temperature water. Do not use tap water as the chlorine and other contaminants can kill the bacteria. If small children won't drink them in water (try giving them a straw to use), you can mix them in apple or pear juice, or, yoghurt (flavored or plain) or applesauce. Just make sure the food/beverage is cool or room-temperature. Only buy probiotic powders that are kept in a refrigerator in the store and then refrigerate them at home - this ensures the bacteria are kept alive and fresh.

Take your first dose of probiotic (follow label instructions for amounts) first thing in the morning and then follow it with some food half an hour later. Take your second dose right before you go to bed at night (on an empty stomach). This will give the bacteria a chance to colonize and really establish themselves while you sleep. Continue this supplementation program throughout the transition from elemental shakes to solids and for two full months after you're eating completely solid foods.

After you've finished your two months of supplementing with Natren brand probiotics, you may want to start on another pro-biotic product called Primal Defense (www.gardenoflifeusa.com). Supplement according to the instructions on the bottle (detailed dosage instructions are available on their website) for 1-3 months and then just take it as needed for maintenance. Primal Defense is a mix of 14 different probiotic strains in a form called Homeostatic Soil Organisms (HSOs). They're different from the Natren probi-otics in that these HSOs are specially cultured in a natural plant substrate that makes them resistant to heat, cold, stomach acids and ascorbic acid. Therefore, the product doesn't need to be refrigerated and the nutrient-rich substrate contains vitamins, minerals, enzymes, proteins, phytonutrients and plant sterols (immune system modulators) which, along with the probiotics, form the proper environment for nutrient absorption and a balanced pH in your intestinal tract. It also contains the probiotic Saccharomyces Boulardii, which has been shown in clinical trials to be particularly beneficial to people with Ulcerative Colitis and Crohn's Disease. Go to their website and click on Jordan's Story - it tells the fascinating story of the formulator of Primal Defense and how he came up with the product.

However, I don't recommend you begin Primal Defense until after you've finished the complete course of Natren probiotics. The Natren probiotics are very gentle on the system with a very low risk of adverse reactions. The Primal Defense product is a more aggressive product (in my opinion), with a variety of new ingredients, and therefore carries a higher risk of adverse reactions like diarrhea or allergies. So it's best to let your body adjust to its newfound state of health and absorption and settle down for a while before introducing an effective product like Primal Defense. If you have a very sensitive system, then you may want to give yourself three to six months of stability before starting the Primal Defense.

Once you've started the probiotic supplementation, do not take antibiotics or have any kind of intestinal exploratory procedure done (colonoscopy, barium enema, etc.) as this will completely disrupt and possibly eliminate the healthy bacterial environment you are trying to establish. If you do have one of these procedures done, try to schedule it before you even start the IBD Remission Diet, or, once you've finished the procedure, or course of antibiotics, begin again with the full program of probiotic supplementation for the full two months. It should be a standard medical procedure to follow any disruption of intestinal flora with probiotic supplementation and although many doctors are now aware of this, it has yet to become an automatic process.

The probiotic powders are also useful to have on hand for any family members who experience a bout of vomiting or diarrhea from travelling, moldy food, bad water, etc. My son Oscar once ate grass from a neighbourhood park while playing football with his Dad. Unfortunately there is a high concentration of dogs in our neighbourhood who all defecate in this park and he must have eaten some dog poop residue. He vomited that night at about 2:00 am and then had diarrhea the next day. I gave him one dose of the three Natren probiotic powders mixed into his yoghurt that evening and by the following day he had one bowel movement in the morning that was semi-formed and then a second that evening that was completely normal. I didn't even need to give him a second dose of probiotics, his bowel movements were normal thereafter.

ONGOING HEALTH

For those of you who don't have my first book, *LISTEN TO YOUR GUT* (www.caramal.com), I'm going to include the Maintenance Diet here from that book. Now that you've restored your intestinal health and gut flora, keep it that way by eating foods and beverages that support your newfound health - not degrade it. This Maintenance Diet should become your normal, natural way of eating for both yourself and your children (give them the best chance of avoiding their genetic predisposition to IBD/IBS):

Maintenance Diet

Make it part of your lifestyle, or second-nature, to adhere to the following as much as possible.

Avoid:

- Alcohol - highly acidic and irritating, but for those times when you must have alcohol, it's my feeling that red wine and Guinness or stout beer are the best forms. If you're okay with milk, it might work well to have Bailey's or Kahlua mixed with milk as milk can coat the stomach and prevent absorption/irritation.

- Caffeine - it inhibits absorption of vitamin C, leaches calcium, magnesium, potassium, iron and trace minerals from the body. Coffee is the worst thing you could drink, really aggravates the colon in particular. Even de-caffeinated coffee is not tolerated well. Bambu is an excellent-tasting Swiss coffee substitute (available on-line or at your local organic store). Pure hot chocolate may be okay, but make it with 3/4 water and only 1/4 milk, or just a little cream.

- Carbonated drinks - you certainly don't need more gas, sugar or caffeine in your system. Also, the carbonation pulls key minerals from your bones like calcium and magnesium.
- Anything containing MSG (interferes with neural functioning) or carrageenan (used in large quantities to induce Ulcerative Colitis in guinea pigs and primates).
- Margarine or butter substitutes - treated with chemical solvents and bleaches, resulting in deformed, highly toxic, trans-fatty acids.
- Hot chillies or peppers.
- Cigarette/cigar/pipe smoke (first or secondhand).
- Artificial sweeteners of any kind (includes aspartame, acesulfame-K, sucralose/splenda, saccharine, etc.) - toxic and proven to cause memory loss, these can also be highly addictive and cause seizures and hyperactivity in some people. If you need an alternative to sugar, use Stevia - a natural herb that is 200-300 times sweeter than sugar, available at health stores.
- Keep processed foods, or foods containing preservatives, nitrates, chemicals, etc. to a minimum or, ideally, completely eliminate them.
- Never use a microwave - damages food at the molecular level, rendering it toxic to your cells and DNA.

Do:

- Use an extra-virgin or virgin olive oil wherever oil is called for in cooking, salads, etc. Cold-pressed oils are superior in retaining nutritional value and are very healthy. Cold-pressed sesame, almond, hemp seed and flax seed oil are also good - basically anything other than mass-market vegetable oils. During the processing of commercial vegetable oils, they are heated to the point where the molecular structure is altered (similar to margarine) resulting in trans-fatty acids that damage cell walls and DNA, and are suspected carcinogens.
- Try to eat fruit in isolation until you've been healed for a year or so and then experiment with mixing it with other foods.

- Reduce milk/milk products. Try to use low-fat Lactaid, rice, goat or almond milk, and certified organic skim-milk yoghurt (fortified with acidophilus and bifidus bacteria). Again, after you've been healed for about a year or so, you'll probably be able to drink regular milk in small quantities or from time to time. Many people find cream (certified organic with no carrageenan or other thickeners added) to be better tolerated than milk. Ideally, only eat cheese made from raw milk (not pasteurized).

- Don't drink milk or juice with meals. If you must have something to drink with your meal, limit yourself to ½ glass of warm or room temperature water, sipped slowly, or a packet of Emergen-C (natural flavored Vitamin C powder) dissolved in ½ glass of water, and then no liquids for an hour after you've eaten. Liquids will interfere with your digestive juices and cause bloating.

- Eat certified organic food and beverages as much as possible.

Following these guidelines, along with maintaining a healthy bacterial flora in your gut, will go a long way to keeping you healthy and energetic. However, if the stressors in your life get to be too much, or you suffer a crisis that results in another flare-up of your condition, keep in mind that you can always go back on the IBD Remission Diet to nurture your body and give it the chance to heal again. The good news is that it's much easier the second time as you already know what to do and are comfortable and familiar with the process. It's also easier because the 'fear factor' isn't present. You'll know the IBD Remission Diet works no matter how bad your bleeding or symptoms are and you'll know you can gain the weight (via good nutrition) needed to heal your body and restore your energy. You'll also get back to eating solids much more quickly, since you won't have to go through the time-consuming process of food allergy/intolerance testing.

EMOTIONAL HEALING

Full and complete healing will also involve addressing the emotional component of your IBD/IBS. All gut disorders are strongly linked to the emotions and some medical researchers have called the gut 'the second brain'. In fact 60% of the body's neurotransmitters are not found in the brain, but rather, in the gastrointestinal tract. Research has also shown that it's not just the brain that can direct or control the gut, but also vice-versa. Certain conditions in the gut can cause depression, for example, in the brain. Many emotions, such as anger and fear, are stored in the gut and even our common language reflects this: "Her stomach twisted in fear" or "His stomach clenched in anger", for example.

If you have IBD or IBS or even just chronic diarrhea or constipation, I can practically guarantee you there are emotional roots to these conditions. If you examine and resolve these root issues or woundings within yourself, you will also see substantial improvement in your physical body. There are many ways to go about this healing and some really effective methods include; hypnotherapy, craniosacral therapy, spiritual or energy healing, and communal prayer or laying-on-of-hands. Psychotherapy or talk-therapy alone are not very effective because they don't integrate with the physical body. Whatever your emotional issues are, they need to be released from your body as well as your mind, so choose a therapy like the ones listed above that facilitates integrated mind/body healing. Dr. Michael Greenwood (see his book listing in Appendix B) sums this up nicely:

> *"I no longer believe in listening to endless stories of victimization. Somewhere along the line, we become the architects of our experience, and by loitering in our own story we perpetuate any illness we might have. Talking is fine for a while, and everyone needs to have their story heard by a sympathetic ear, but there comes a time we must get into the body if we want to heal the body." (pg. 296, Braving The Void)*

Please see Appendix B for a recommended reading list of books I've found particularly helpful or illuminating in this area of healing.

EXERCISE TO INCREASE & MAINTAIN HEALTH

I've been physically active playing numerous sports, skiing, horseriding, training martial arts, etc. throughout my life. However, I've found that for foundational health, no matter how weak and sick you are, nothing beats weight training. Vigorous exercise can often result in a suppression of the immune system, so for someone whose immune system is already not functioning well, a strenuous exercise session can leave you feeling quite sick.

Weight training, however, is an ideal form of exercise because it can be easily adapted to fit your personal goals and needs. It can be an aerobic workout, or, it can be a slow-paced, calm activity with lots of rest periods. You can weight train to give yourself a toned, stream-lined appearance, or, you can use it to bulk up and increase your muscle size dramatically. It is also the best method of promoting weight gain for people who are malnourished or underweight. If you want to gain weight, you have to create a demand in your body for additional muscle. Lying down or sitting all day does not require your body to produce extra muscle fibre, while weight training does. Lastly, numerous studies have shown it to be a great defence against osteoporosis as it strengthens bones and increases their density. If you've been on steroids (eg. Prednisone) for any length of time, you should definitely weight train as a preventative against osteoporosis and also to help repair the damage caused by the steroids.

When you should begin your weight training program depends on how weak you are when you start the IBD Remission Diet. If you're 99 pounds, have been haemorrhaging, and find it hard to get out of bed when you first start the Diet, then wait until you're up to 107 pounds (for example) and can walk a block or two. This may sound too weak/sick to begin, but trust me, as long as you proceed slowly and stay in touch with your body throughout the session, you'll heal much faster by beginning to exercise sooner. The first few times you go to the gym, you may only do one set of very light weights for 10 or 15 minutes total. That's great! As long as you go

2-3 times/week, whatever you manage to do is great. But, do not exercise to exhaustion. You can leave the gym feeling tired, but you shouldn't feel exhausted or completely worn out - if you do, you've done too much and it will be counter-productive.

For the first three weeks I was on the elemental diet (the first time) I couldn't do more than walk around my apartment. I gradually increased this to walking 20 feet up and down the sidewalk outside - getting fresh air is really important - with someone there in case I needed support or felt faint. I then increased this gradually to a block or two and when I could walk three blocks, I had my husband drive me to the gym. My first time at the gym, I could only manage one set each of only three different exercises, and between each set I lay down on the mats for 5-10 minutes and just rested, stretching my arms out above my head. Then my husband drove me home. I had to start very slowly as I'd had severe haemorrhaging that had really weakened my body.

This may all sound rather unimpressive, but, by doing these little bits of exercise and gradually increasing each day, by the end of seven weeks I was riding my bike and doing regular workouts at the gym, 35 pounds heavier and healthy in every way. Six weeks later I was pregnant with my son Oscar (who also enjoys superb health and energy).

You need to exercise the following muscle groups to get a good, full body workout and to create the demand for your body to gain healthy, solid weight:

- Biceps (the large bulging muscle on the upper front part of your arm)
- Triceps (the opposing smaller muscle on the upper back part of your arm)
- Quadriceps (also known as the thigh muscle)
- Hamstrings (the back of the thigh)
- Calves
- Abdominals (working these muscles will also strengthen your lower back)

If you're not familiar with weight training, just take this list of muscle groups to an instructor at your gym and have them show you the machines or free weights you can use to exercise each one. Do two sets of each exercise, with 10 repetitions of the exercise per set. I like to do just one set of each muscle group and then do the whole circuit again a second time. For example, rather than doing two sets of bicep curls in a row, I'll do:

- one set of 10 bicep curls
- one set of 10 tricep extensions
- one set of 10 leg extensions (quadriceps)
- one set of 10 leg presses (also quads)
- one set of 10 hamstring curls
- one set of 10 calf raises
- one set of 25 crunches (abdominals).

I'll then start all over again at the beginning of that sequence and do the second set of each exercise. This gives each muscle group a chance to rest while you're working the other muscles. To establish the amount of weight you should lift with each exercise, experiment until you find the amount of weight that makes it really hard to complete the tenth repetition of the exercise. This indicates the right threshold for your body. When it becomes easy to perform the tenth repetition, you need to increase the threshold. You can do this by either increasing the number of repetitions (up to 60 repetitions per set), or by leaving the reps the same and increasing the amount of weight you're lifting. Increasing the repetitions of each exercise will result in lean, streamlined muscles. Increasing the weight lifted per exercise will result in bigger, bulkier muscle, so do whichever meets your personal goals or preference for your body.

It's also really important to stretch your body out after exercising it so your muscles don't get tense or crampy. Stretching or yoga is wonderful for improving circulation, blood flow and toxin flushing. Do at least 10 minutes of stretching following your weight training routine. Again, if you don't know any stretches, ask an instructor at the gym to show you a simple routine. Many gyms have posters with all the stretches illustrated so you can follow the figures each time in case you forget between workouts. Sometimes I'll stretch out certain muscles between exercises and then at the end of both sets I like to do about 20-30 minutes of continuous stretching.

Again, when you're first beginning, start out really slowly and if all you can do is a few of the exercises, then that's great! You may also want to proceed slowly with the abdominal exercises as your tummy area is likely to be quite tender - just start with 3-5 crunches to begin with and increase as it feels comfortable. Putting in the effort to learn weight training will pay dividends for the rest of your life. It's an ideal form of exercise that can be used whether you're healthy, ill, pregnant, injured or elderly - again, because weight training increases bone density, it's a particularly ideal workout for people aged 50 and older, or those at risk of osteoporosis.

TAKE ACTION

Spend some time thinking about the possible emotional roots or contributors to your dis-ease. What type of integrated body/mind therapy do you think would best help you at this time:

_____

_____

_____

_____

Make a list of potential therapists you could go and explore your healing with, include a craniosacral therapist, a hypnotherapist, and an energy or spiritual healer you've heard good things about (include their phone numbers here for easy reference):

_____

_____

_____

_____

What are you going to do to increase your muscular and cardiovascular health? List a gym or two you can go and check out to see if you like the atmosphere. Also list the phone number and address of your community center and see if they have facilities for weight training:

_____

_____

_____

_____

_____

If there's no way you'll ever work out at a gym, list a program of home exercises you can do, or a videotape you could get to do in your living room that incorporates some type of weight-bearing activity (either your own body weight, hand weights, or rubber tubing):

_____

_____

_____

_____

_____

_____

Or, what about a yoga studio nearby? List the address and phone number of one or two you'd like to try:

_____

_____

6

SUMMARY
& ACTION PLAN

*B*efore everything else, getting ready is the secret of success.
Henry Ford

Y OU SHOULD NOW HAVE a complete overview of the IBD Remission Diet along with detailed instructions and hopefully you're feeling pretty confident about embarking on it. But just to pull things together and make it really easy, here's a step-by-step plan of action to help you implement the IBD Remission Diet:

TIMELINE & CHECKLIST

☐ Figure out how long you need to go on the elemental diet for and how many shakes per day you'll need to consume to meet your calorie requirements. Don't forget that as your weight increases, so does your calorie and protein requirement.

☐ Order in enough Absorb Plus (or ingredients to mix your own) to last you the duration of the Diet, or at least to give you enough lead time before you need to place another order and wait for mail/courier delivery. Contact www.absorbplus.com or 1-800-460-8606 to order Absorb Plus, or inquire about shipping times.

☐ Order your supply of MucosaHeal (www.mucosaheal.com or toll-free: 1-800-550-9659) and order any FissureHeal suppositories you may need at the same time to save on shipping, as both are made by the same company.

☐ Go to a health store and purchase the following supplements:
   • Coenzyme Q10 (30 mg. capsules)★
   • Pycnogenol (30 mg. capsules)★
   • Vitamin C in mineral ascorbate (calcium ascorbate, magnesium ascorbate etc.) powder form
   • Ferrasorb Iron (by Thorne Research, 25 mg. capsules)★ - if anemic
   • Mixed Bioflavonoids (each capsule containing approx. 50 mg. each of Rutin, Quercetin, Hesperidin)★
   • George's Roadrunner Aloe Vera Juice
   • Spectrum Naturals cold-pressed organic flax oil, and/or,

Udo's Choice Perfected Oil Blend. Get a small bottle and keep refrigerated.

make sure you get capsules, not tablets, as you need to open them and empty the contents into the shakes.

☐ Decide which broths you want to make and purchase the necessary certified organic meat and/or vegetables. If you like, make them up now and freeze them in individual servings in ziplock freezer bags to use as needed. Buy a blender (ideally with a glass jar) if you don't have one, to whip the shakes.

☐ Schedule time off work or some kind of extra help for when you first start the Diet so you give yourself time and space to make all the changes and get used to eating this way. Also schedule a massage or relaxing spa appointment. Massage will further stimulate blood flow and the release and flushing of toxins from your body, so try to have one per week, whilst on the IBD Remission Diet, if possible.

☐ Okay, time to start the elemental diet! Whip up your first shake:

IBD Remission Diet Shake Recipe with Supplements
1. Pour one cup (8 oz) of cold or room-temperature spring or filtered water into a blender

2. Add 1 serving of Absorb Plus (100 grams/4 level scoops)

3. Add the supplements of your choice:
   • Alternate Coenzyme Q10 (30 mg. per shake) with Pycnogenol (30 mg. per shake) i.e. put CoQ10 in one shake, then Pycnogenol in the next and so on. To a combined maximum of 200 mg. per day.
   • Vitamin C in mineral ascorbate (calcium ascorbate, magnesium ascorbate etc.) form (1000 mg. per shake, to a maximum of 10,000 mg. per day)
   • Iron - if anemic (1 capsule/25 mg. 1-2 times per day, ferrous citrate is the best form of iron)

- Mixed Bioflavonoids containing approx. 50 mg. each of Rutin, Quercetin, Hesperidin (1 capsule per shake to a maximum of 6 capsules per day)

4. Add 1 tsp. - 1 tbsp. of organic flax or Udo's oil (according to tolerance, to a maximum of 8 tablespoons per day)

5. Whip on high speed for 10-15 seconds

6. Pour into a glass over ice, drink through a straw, and enjoy!

Alternate these shakes with broths and plenty of filtered or spring water, along with the other allowable snacks. Enjoy the experience of renewed health and good solid weight that is gradually building up in your body.

☐ Take your other supplements between shakes, on an empty stomach, as needed: George's Aloe Vera Juice and MucosaHeal. Use the FissureHeal suppositories at night to heal any anal/rectal fissures you might have.

☐ As soon as you're able, begin weight training at your local gym. Start slowly and don't exhaust yourself.

☐ As your time on the elemental diet draws to a close, go to the health store and buy your probiotics. Either Natren's Trenev (if you can swallow pills) or Natren's Mega Dophilus, Bifido Factor and Digesta Lac powders that you can mix together in water (or yoghurt or apple juice for kids).

☐ Follow the FOOD REINTRODUCTION CHART as you begin to eat solids again and simultaneously begin probiotic supplementation. Keep a food journal (or photocopy the one on page 98-99) of foods and physical reactions, emotional feelings, etc.

☐ Once you're completely on solid foods, continue probiotic supplementation for an additional two months and follow the MAINTENANCE DIET as part of your regular way of eating.

☐ Line up some appointments for emotional, mind/body healing, like craniosacral therapy, hypnotherapy, or energy or spiritual healing.

☐ Once you've finished the complete course of Natren probiotics and you're feeling really settled into your new-found state of health (anywhere from three to six months after completing the elemental diet), begin supplementing with Primal Defense to further enhance your intestinal environment, digestion and immune system.

Although following the IBD Remission Diet may seem tedious and difficult, keep in mind that upon completion you'll also have given yourself the gift of peace. You'll most likely have a deep sense of peace and absence of fear, with the assurance that no matter how bad it gets, you now have a tool you can use to heal yourself quickly and naturally. You may find you no longer live with the fear of emergency admittance to the hospital, no more threat of TPN or stomach shunt tubes, or surgery, or damaging drugs. Although six weeks without solid food may seem too difficult to embark on, put it in perspective. What is your life like now? How bad is your day-to-day existence and how long has it been this bad for? Do you really want to go through years more of this fear, pain and ugliness, when only six weeks could completely change your life? Just imagine what it would be like to have enough energy to get through a day, to be able to laugh and run and jump and enjoy mealtimes again. Imagine what it would be like to travel and have adventures and not even think about doctors and hospitals. Yes, it is possible! Whatever difficulties you experience following the IBD Remission Diet, you will be so well rewarded. It is a fantastic, completely natural way to achieve long-term health and peace for your body. And surely, that's the greatest gift you could give yourself.

PRACTICAL QUESTIONS & ANSWERS

Q I assume it's okay to use vegetables other than the ones you list in your recipe for veggie broth in the book. I'd like to use celery and onions, but maybe the latter would be too harsh? I also drank the store-bought vegetable broth (it's Imagine brand, which you probably know). Was somewhat concerned that it is quite opaque. No bits floating anywhere, but is this okay do you think?

A Yes, you can use whatever veggies you like in the homemade vegetable broth, it's just a matter of taste preference. What does the ingredient list on the store-bought vegetable broth say? If there is any added starch or thickeners, it's not okay. Also, call the company and check with them whether it contains pureed vegetables or just the liquid and ask them why it's opaque. Pureed vegetables are not okay. If it's not clear, it probably contains some sort of added ingredient or pulp residue and that's not okay on the elemental diet.

Q My husband says he doesn't want to use the oils in his shakes because he doesn't want the extra calories. He wants to LOSE 10 lbs over the 2 weeks on the elemental diet if he can. Do you think this is reasonable? Seems to me the oil is part of the therapy as well.

A Yes, the oil is definitely a beneficial part of the therapy and this kind of oil (flax, Udo's, etc.) doesn't get converted to fat - it's used for many other vital (often deficient) things in the body. But he could drop it to ½ tbsp. oil per shake (that would still give him a good daily dose) and then just monitor the overall calorie count accordingly. Remember that with any diet if you lose too much weight too quickly it just slows down the body's metabolism and when you eat regular food again, you'll just put on more weight than you lost, because now your metabolism's slower. I would recommend he maintain a decent caloric intake and add some exercise. Go power walking or jogging, or just do pushups, situps, squats, etc. in the house if he can't get to the gym - anything that produces a sweat is a sufficient workout to raise metabolism and therefore burn up some fat.

Q   I had my first elemental bowel movement today. I had to run to the bathroom and it was all dark, scary looking liquid with tiny black particles (like ground pepper) floating in it. Is that from the Absorb Plus Chocolate Royale flavor, perhaps? Do you think that as my bowel heals that this urgency will go away or is it because the stool is liquid that it's that much harder to hold (obviously, I have this problem anyway, so it's hard to differentiate)?

A   The black particles could be from the Chocolate Royale, or they could be something already in your colon that's being flushed out. You may see a lot of weird stuff in your bowel movements since you're on an exclusively elemental diet, which is also an automatic cleanse and detox. You may even see solid bits of stool at some point amidst the liquid and this could be impacted fecal matter that's been stuck in the folds of your intestine for months or years. If you see pink or red liquid, don't be alarmed, that's the natural color from the Mixed Berry coming through. Again, because your fecal matter is completely liquid, everything is visible. Liquid bowel movements are also definitely much more urgent and harder to hold than solid. Again, this is normal and may or may not lessen in urgency as the diet progresses.

Q   I read what you wrote about drinking the Absorb Plus shakes slowly over 15-30 minutes. But I can't seem to stop from glugging the whole thing back in 5 minutes. Is this bad?

A   The reason you're advised to drink it slowly is: because Absorb Plus is pre-digested, it hits your bloodstream very quickly and this can either give people a 'sugar high' followed by a mood/sleepy crash, or, make them nauseous. If you're not having any problems drinking it quickly then it's ok, you're still getting the same nutrients. Oh yes, except if you're adding Vitamin C - that's best absorbed when drunk slowly. If you drink it fast then you'll just pee out a lot of the Vitamin C because your body can't absorb it quickly enough. Try to stretch it to 15 minutes ideally, at least.

Reader comment on mixing Absorb Plus:

It took a few tries to figure out the best way to blend the shakes. I found that when I followed the instructions and put the water in first and the powder second that I was left with big globs of powder at the bottom of the drinks and also on the side of the blender. What seems to work perfectly is putting the powder and supplements in first, then the oil, then the water. I blend it and then re-blend for a briefer period to crush in some ice. This leaves no sludge and the drinks really do taste great. No gagging them back at all. Clearly the colder they are, the better.

Response:

It must depend on the type of blender you have which way works better - good thing you've worked it out and thanks for letting me know. I'm glad you find the taste as good as I do - especially when you've had to drink the other stuff out there!

Q How long exactly does it take for all the bacteria in the colon to die off once you're on the elemental diet?

A That's a very good question and not even the scientists nor gastroenterologists I've talked to know the answer. The common length of time prescribed by doctors to be on the elemental diet is six weeks, so maybe that facilitates complete clearing of the bacterial flora. However, when I went on the elemental diet for two weeks I saw beneficial results, so even that length of time must alter the flora significantly. If you ever find out, please let me know!

Q Can I add other supplements (other than the ones you've listed) to the shakes?

A Yes, as long as they're in elemental form. If they're plant products like spirulina, algae, etc., they're complex carbohydrates and not allowed. All carbohydrates must be in monosaccharide form so they're absorbed directly into the bloodstream and don't require digestion. Other oils are fine as long as they're cold-pressed and preferably certified organic. If you're unsure about something, either check with the manufacturer, or don't add it!

Q Well it's the end of day six on the elemental diet and for some reason I had mild stomach cramps all day. Just felt a bit out of sorts and very tired at day's end too. I think I may be close to ovulating, so it could be related, but surely if the drinks didn't agree with me I'd have bigger problems by now? Just wondering if you ever experienced stuff like this? Also, my husband says he just hasn't felt all that great since he's been on the diet. Like he's looking at the world through a fog. He's also been very tired at night and has had a few headaches. Could this just be detox, do you think? He says he was drinking an average of one cup of tea and three cups of coffee a day before the diet so his withdrawal shouldn't be that bad. Just thought I'd bounce this off you. Of course, we could both have a bug, and I am a bit anemic right now. I do instinctively feel that colon-wise things are improving. Only because I don't wake up in the morning tripping over myself to get to the bathroom. Things feel a little more under control. What do you think?

A Try not to micro-examine things too much as symptoms and feelings will come and go for a variety of reasons and some days will be better than others - just like life! The food clearing literature I've read says that people can experience withdrawal/clearing symptoms for 10-14 days, so that may be what's happening with your husband. Also, is he consuming enough calories, because that could make him tired and foggy too? Especially if he's trying to maintain his normal schedule and activity level, because don't forget, as the shakes are pre-digested, they hit the bloodstream very quickly and then there's no sustained release of nutrients/energy as there is with normal food. So you can feel tired or a bit weak within 45 minutes of drinking one - especially if he's drinking them down quickly. If you're resting a lot and taking it easy, you won't notice this so much, but if you're running around living your normal life I'm sure you'd feel weaker and more fuzzy than normal (also due to quickly fluctuating blood sugar levels as, again, the shakes hit the bloodstream quite quickly compared to normal food).

Remember too that the IBD Remission Diet is a whole program and everyone responds differently. You may not feel the full benefits of the program until you've started regular food and probiotics again - and then the foundation you've been laying down during this period becomes evident. Try to hang in there and just listen to your body. Do the relaxation and getting in touch with your gut/intuition exercise again if you have questions you want answered by your body.

Q What's the best way to mix the shakes when I'm away from home?

A Well here's an excellent answer direct from one of my readers: "I've been making my shakes at work using a Braun hand blender. I keep a small bottle of oil and some spring water ice in the fridge/freezer there, and take a thermos of broth with me every day. I find the consistency of the shakes using the hand blender is particularly frothy and good. Anyway, just thought this might be useful info. for anyone attempting to do the elemental diet who's worrying about carting in a giant blender to their workplace everyday."

Of course, if you're not adding oil to the shakes, you can just follow the directions on the jar of Absorb Plus and mix them by hand with a spoon. You can pre-measure a single serving of Absorb

Plus into a zip-lock bag and bring any capsules etc. you need to add in another zip-lock bag. If you're adding additional supplements though, you'll need to whip the shake with some kind of hand-held blender to get everything to mix properly - and maybe whip again once or twice while drinking it. Even a little bit of oil makes a big difference as it will hold the supplements in suspension and keep them from settling immediately on the bottom of the glass. If you have no access to a fridge, then pack capsules of flax oil in a bag or thermos of ice, when you make your shake, just puncture the capsules and squeeze the oil into the shake mixture.

Q Since you formulated Absorb Plus, do you benefit financially from sales of the product?

A For Absorb Plus (and any other products I formulate) I charge a one-time formulation fee, which I am paid regardless of whether the product sells, or not. The product formula is also protected in that the company cannot change the formula (eg. use cheaper ingredients, add artificial ingredients, etc.) without my consent - this ensures the integrity and quality standards of the product I formulated are maintained.

Q Can I use Absorb Plus with my stomach shunt tube and have it pumped directly into my stomach rather than swallowing it?

A The company that makes Absorb Plus has not done any tests on having the product directly pumped into the stomach. However, I have heard from a reader who used it this way with no problems, and also the ingredient profile (in terms of its degree of elemental components) is similar to the hospital products recommended for this purpose. As equipment changes, the best thing is to let your gastroenterologist or IBD nurse have a look at Absorb Plus to determine if it's compatible with your pump and tubing apparatus. Also, double-check whether you can add all the recommended supplements as well.

Q I'm nearly finished the elemental diet and am feeling quite anxious about eating regular food again. I'm really worried about what will happen and also I've felt so good on the diet I almost wish I could just drink the shakes and forget about food. The other thing is the thought of all that shopping, cooking, cleaning the kitchen, etc. is really not appealing - it's been so quick and easy to eat this way. Do you think I'm odd?

A No, it's perfectly normal to feel all of those things. When food has made you feel uncomfortable or ill for so long, then you find something that nourishes you and makes you feel good, it's only natural to want to stick with it. Your anxiety is also completely understandable - don't judge yourself, just allow the feelings to come, and allow them to go, and keep moving forward, step by step. I still have an Absorb Plus shake occasionally when I don't feel like cooking, or don't have much appetite, so don't worry as that option is always available!

Q Should I continue taking the antioxidants when I come off the shakes? I don't want to end up in a situation where I'm taking a million supplements four times a day because it always drives me crazy and then I tend to give everything up. So I will need to prioritize... Also, I'm planning on getting pregnant as soon as possible, so what do you advise in that instance?

A Regarding continued supplementation, I know what you mean and my definition of health is NOT having to consume 50 different supplements every day for the rest of your life! My advice would be twofold: Firstly, identify your particular health priorities and therefore the supplements that will benefit you the most/are most needed by your body. Then, take just those supplements once a day (mornings for example) and make it a routine.

That's why I suggest you may want to continue taking a shake per day (easiest is to have one instead of breakfast) as it's such an easy way to take the flax oil and supplements. However, you could also just swallow the supplements along with your normal breakfast and swallow the oil in capsule form and/or try to work it into your normal diet (salad dressings, drizzled over vegetables - let them cool down first though, etc.). Since you're planning on getting pregnant, you definitely want to continue with the flax oil (or Udo's) as it's particularly vital for fetal brain development in the first and third trimester - one to two tablespoons per day is sufficient.

Secondly, (if you're not pregnant) I would then cycle one month ON - taking all the supplements every day, and then one month OFF - no supplements. I believe this actually enhances absorption and utilisation of supplements as the body doesn't adjust to anything long-term. Remember one of the strongest principles of the body is the homeostatic mechanism. Therefore, I believe if you take a substance continually, long-term, the body will simply adjust to that intake and either reduce its own production of that substance, or, extract less from your food. Of course there are many distinguished proponents of natural health who would strongly disagree with me, so keep in mind this is just my opinion and you should follow your own convictions/intuition on this issue. Of course, if you're in a disease-state, you need ongoing, continual supplementation until your deficiencies are addressed. But, once you've reached a state of health (balance) I see no reason to continue the same volume and frequency of supplementation.

So, for my personal advice on which supplements you should continue taking once you're finished the IBD Remission Diet and have achieved a state of health/balance, I would recommend the following daily (and then cycling on/off each month):

- full-spectrum multi-vitamin (with high levels of Vit.B complex and Vit.E)
- full-spectrum multi-mineral (including trace minerals as well)
- 1-2 tbsp. flax or Udo's oil per day (or fish oil capsules if you prefer - but make sure they're tested for toxicity)

- 1-3, 1000 mg. packets of flavored Emergen-C (Vitamin C ascorbates) per day - if you take it in this form it doesn't feel like a chore, but rather a treat; a nice fizzy drink with ice that tastes really good.

If you're pregnant, I would continue on this regimen uninterrupted (no cycling on/off) throughout the pregnancy and breastfeeding. If your baby gets sick, you can bump up to as much as 10,000 mg. Vitamin C per day and also take some Astragalus (liquid tincture from Herb Pharm, 20 drops in a bit of warm water 1-3x/day is best), both of these will go straight through to the breastmilk and baby will be cured very, very quickly. However, if baby's running a high fever, don't take the Astragalus (it can encourage sweating) but just the mega-doses of Vitamin C in mineral ascorbate form.

If your diet consists of mostly certified organic food, then after 6 months to a year of this supplementation, you may wish to take the supplements listed above only when your body tells you it needs them, or when you get run down, flu season, etc. Also, remember to take probiotics as needed (whenever your stool gets too runny or too hard or you tend toward diarrhea or constipation).

Q I'm feeling kind of worried now, I had one bout of definite diarrhea late this afternoon (but not much quantity as I've hardly eaten anything). Now I notice I'm starting to get tender red bumps on my legs, similar to when I had a reaction to Asacol (there's only about 3-4 bumps so far). What do I do now? Go back on the elemental diet for another week? The only potentially allergenic thing I can think that I've eaten so far is that the first squash I had yesterday only had olive oil and salt on it. Then, the second time I had it in the afternoon I put butter and salt on it. I could lay off the butter and see if that helps. Any suggestions?

A Yes, from what you've told me, the most likely culprit is probably the butter. However, only your body knows whether you need to stay on the diet longer or if you're reacting to a food, and which one. I suggest you don't consume any butter for a week or two - until the red bumps are completely clear and then eat a nice big amount of it again and see what happens. If nothing, eat it again 2-3 times (keeping all else the same) and if still nothing, then it probably wasn't butter, but if it is, you should get a reaction fairly quickly again.

Remember too, that food intolerances have thresholds - once a week may be fine, but three times a week may trigger a reaction. You're just going to have to test and re-test. You could also find a naturopath who does Vega Testing for food allergies and see what the correlations are. If possible find a clinic that also has a 'desensitization' program where they use homeopathic remedies to desensitize you to those foods if you wish.

I wouldn't worry so much about diarrhea at this stage because as long as your food source is primarily elemental, you're going to have urgent, liquid bowel movements and it can also take a while for the probiotics to build up enough to firm up your stool. The red bumps do indicate a reaction though, and that's what you want to pinpoint the cause of. At any rate, try to calm down and get in touch with your intuition - all the answers are within you and if you access that wisdom you'll get your answers much faster than the time-consuming process of scientific trial-testing.

Also, strongly consider using this time to get into the body-emotional connections/triggers you may have. Remember all illness is not just a physical phenomenon and if we don't heal the emotional we'll keep having the physical recur.Hypnotherapy and craniosacral or energy/spiritual healing are all good modalities for healing body-located emotional roots.

Q It's day six of my food reintroduction program and I ate a chicken breast roasted in olive oil and salt and it produced no reaction and NO STOOL. Is this normal? A friend had warned me about this from what he'd observed in hospital, that it's pretty well all water, so no food waste came out at all. Yesterday I had rice cooked in broth for lunch and then a pretty full meal of rice, tuna and zucchini for dinner (bad food combining, I guess, but it seemed like the right thing). So far, so good. I did have one bowel movement first thing this morning, which was small and runny, but digested and still affected by the two shakes I also had yesterday. No bloating, or gas, or gastric discomfort. Overall I feel really good. Did an intensive yoga class two nights ago that would have been unimaginable a couple of months ago. My skin looks better than usual and my energy is great. So I feel positive. I'll try not to worry about the diarrhea thing and hope it will take care of itself once I'm totally back on solids.

A Remember too that healthy digestion means food takes between 24-48 hours to transit to fecal matter so that chicken may still be on its way out yet. Also, it's not just the solid food intake that remedies the diarrhea, it's the re-population and build up of good bacterial flora that's primarily responsible for that, so you have to allow some time for that colonization to take place. And of course, the time that takes is going to vary from person to person. I think your rice, tuna, zucchini meal is good food combining (many proponents of food combining find they can tolerate rice with protein) and the perfect type of meal for where you're at (or anyone really!). If you follow your own body's wisdom - above any rules - you will always do what's best for you at that time.

Q I spent the morning reviewing my food diary looking for some connections which made me feel proactive about things. I looked at days where I was having solid bowel movements and no welts, and thought I should just try to go back to my menu for those two days prior and avoid the items that preceded diarrhea or welts. Obvious, I know. I have been concentrating, as you suggested, on the fact that I feel great. Totally normal. When the diarrhea hits, it's fast, and over fast too, and unlike before it's not making me feel weak or making my guts heave and cramp. So what are your thoughts on the wisdom - if one were having a mini-flare, or sudden return of certain symptoms - of retreating back to shakes for, say, two or three days. Just to keep things in check. Do you think there'd be any benefit or do you think it needs to be a longer chunk of time? My own feeling is that this would keep a symptom from running its course by stopping it in its tracks.

A Yes, if your symptoms are caused by food intolerance/allergy, then going on the shakes for a few days would certainly be an effective clearing therapy. However, if symptoms are caused by a 'disease flare-up' then you need to go back on the elemental diet for at least 3 weeks (many doctors recommend 6 weeks) to give the body a chance to heal properly and thoroughly before introducing food again. But it sounds like your symptoms are food intolerance-related, yes? Follow your own intuition (use the relaxation exercise in Chapter Two) and you'll know what to do.

Q If a food is going to cause gas, within what timeframe do you think it should typically do so? I ate some sautéed green peppers at lunch (12:00). It's now 8.30 pm and I haven't had any gas or discomfort. So do you think I can classify this food as 'safe' in terms of gas/bloating?

A If food causes gas, usually it's anywhere from immediately to within about four hours of eating. Traditionally, carbohydrates take 1-1.5 hours to digest in the stomach and then begin their passage through the intestines, meat takes 2-2.5 hours in the stomach and fruit takes about 15-20 minutes. So, depending on where your gas occurs (stomach, bowels, etc.) and how long after eating it happens, you can narrow down the likely culprits. 8.5 hours and I'd say you're free and clear! Traditional, complete digestion of a food through the entire digestive tract takes 24 - 48 hours (when I use the word 'traditional' here I'm referring to the digestive process in healthy, normal systems) so technically, I guess a food could cause gas up to 48 hours later if the gas was in the colon. However, I've never had such a delayed reaction, nor known of anyone else who has. I think in people with sensitive digestive systems, you'd see bloating or gas pains within four hours - maybe six hours at the outside.

Q I've been doing quite a bit of reading about elemental diets on the web and have found article after article from all over the world (MEDICAL studies) that say what you do: That these diets are as effective as steroids for attaining remission but have the added benefit of actually healing the bowel. So why is this not even mentioned as a possibility by my GI? Clearly because it doesn't sell drugs. I just find the whole thing so blatant.

A Yes, I know what you mean about the elemental diet - I think a lot of GIs (gastroenterologists) don't bother with it because the compliance rate is really low. And if you've tasted the hospital elemental diet products you'll know why! Also, they don't have the yummy broths and jello to help them along - just nauseatingly sweet, thick drinks that contain so much low quality oil they make your guts spasm constantly. In addition, just an elemental diet alone won't provide the level of healing that the IBD Remission Diet does - because of the targeted supplementation plan, probiotic colonization and systematic food reintroduction testing. Well, hopefully this book will be the first step in increasing awareness and facilitating implementation of this wonderful natural healing program for people!

Q The Natren Healthy Trinity probiotic capsules are very expensive. On sale they're $25 for 14 caps. So if I took 2 a day that's like $100 a month! Does this make sense to you? I've been taking probiotics for 3 weeks already, so could I get away with just taking the 1 a day as prescribed on the label?

A Yes, you'll probably be OK with just the one a day at this point. Experiment with taking it 1) first thing in the morning, wait 20 minutes then have breakfast, versus, 2) at night on an empty stomach before bed, and see which way works better. Natren is so expensive because it's a) top of the line and they're one of the few companies to guarantee a certain amount of live bacteria per bottle, b) it contains all 3 strains of probiotics - acidophilus, bifidum and bulgaricus - most other probiotics only contain 2 strains, and c) they use a human strain rather than porcine (pig) or bovine (cow) strain - which most other companies use. Maybe that's why I find it so effective - because they use only human strains of probiotics. If your bowels are doing really well (no diarrhea, etc.) then you may only need to take 1 capsule every other day after the first month. If you can at all afford it, I suggest you stick with the Natren brand probiotics, otherwise, ask your health store for their recommendation as to the next best brand.

I'd love to hear from you! Any comments, questions or stories of your own healing journey are most welcome. It's easiest for me to reply by email, so please include an email address for yourself if possible. You can reach me at:

Email: jini@caramal.com

Or

Jini Patel Thompson
c/o Caramal Publishing Inc.
PO Box 29022
Vancouver, BC V6J 5C2
Canada

Appendix A

PRODUCT SUPPLIER LIST

If you have trouble finding any of the products or supplements mentioned in this book, please contact:

Finlandia Natural Pharmacy

1964 West Broadway,
Vancouver, BC, V6J 1Z2
Canada
toll-free: 1-800-363-4372
tel: 604-733-5323
fax: 604-733-5340
www.finlandiapharmacy.com
You can order most - if not all - of the products listed in this book from Finlandia and they ship worldwide.

Aloe Vera Juice

George's Roadrunner Aloe Vera Juice
Warren Laboratories Inc.
1656 I-35 South Abbott, Texas
76621, USA
www.warrenlabsaloe.com
tel: 254-580-9990
toll-free: 1-800-421-2563
fax: 254-580-9944
Available at reputable health stores and some organic grocery stores.

Cold-Pressed Oils

Spectrum Naturals Inc.
1304 South Point Blvd.
Suite 28, Petaluma
CA, 94954, USA
tel: 707-778-8900
www.spectrumnaturals.com
Available in all organic grocery stores and some regular grocery stores.

Udo's Choice Perfected Oil Blend

www.udoerasmus.com
toll-free: 1-888-436-6697
email questions: lfair@florahealth.com
Available in all health and organic grocery stores.

Elemental Shakes
Absorb Plus
3 Flavors: French Vanilla, Mixed Berry, Chocolate Royale
Imix Naturals Inc.
PO Box 500008, Austin, TX
78750, USA
toll-free: 1-800-460-8606
tel: 512-288-5005
www.absorbplus.com
Not available in retail stores, order on-line or by phone.

Intestinal Healing Formula
MucosaHeal
Ahten Inc.
PO Box 500108
Austin, Texas
78750, USA
toll-free: 1-800-550-9659
www.mucosaheal.com
Not available in retail stores, order on-line or by phone.

Probiotics
Trenev (capsules) OR
Digesta Lac, Bifido Factor & Mega Dophilus (powders)

Natren Inc.
3105 Willow Lane,
Westlake Village, CA
91361, USA
toll-free: 1-800-992-3323
www.natren.com

Available in the refrigerator at reputable health stores and some organic grocery stores.

Primal Defense (available in caplets or powder)
Garden of Life Inc.
1449 Jupiter Park Drive Suite 16
Jupiter, Florida
33458, USA
email questions: customerservice@gardenoflifeusa.com
www.gardenoflifeusa.com
Available through their website and at reputable health stores.

Suppositories
FissureHeal
Ahten Inc.
PO Box 500108
Austin, Texas
78750, USA
toll-free: 1-800-550-9659
www.fissureheal.com
Not available in retail stores, order on-line or by phone.

Vitamin C
Emergen-C
Naturally Flavored Drink Powders (Cranberry, Raspbery, Lemon-Lime, Cola, Tangerine, etc.)
Alacer Corp.
toll-free: 1-800-663-6663
www.alacercorp.com
Available in all health and organic grocery stores.

Appendix **B**

RECOMMENDED READING

Braving The Void by Michael Greenwood, MD
Dr. Greenwood uses acupuncture to access mind/body integration and healing. Acupuncture on the part of the body that is experiencing pain causes the mind/body to enter 'the void' where the root causes of the trauma/illness are brought to consciousness and offered up for healing. The book is filled with fascinating case studies from his practice.
www.gordonsoules.com

Through Time Into Healing: *Discovering the Power of Regression Therapy to Erase Trauma and Transform Mind, Body and Relationships* by Brian L. Weiss, MD
Dr. Weiss is a Yale graduate psychiatrist who uses a form of hypnotherapy called Regression Therapy to help clients access events in their past or past lives that are the source of current pain or illness - and to heal and release these traumas from the mind/body. The book is filled with interesting case studies from his practice.
Simon and Schuster Inc.

Touch of Hope: *The Autobiography of a Laying-On-Of-Hands Healer* by Dean Kraft (with Rochelle Kraft)
A well-written story of the author's discovery and development of his gift, with lots of case studies (stories of actual clients and their healings), scientific scrutiny of his powers, and instructions on how to stimulate and use your own healing ability.
Penguin Putnam Inc.

Why People Don't Heal and How They Can by Caroline Myss
The title says it all; looks at emotional and mental blockages to healing, how they interplay with the physical and what you can do about it.
www.randomhouse.com

Remarkable Healings: *A Psychiatrist Discovers Unsuspected Roots of Mental and Physical Illness* by Shakuntala Modi, MD
Dr. Modi uses hypnotherapy to effect both past life and spiritual healing. A really in-depth, fascinating book that looks at the roots of both physical and emotional trauma, and harmful spirit or energy attachments, and how to release them.
www.hrpub.com

Index

Natren probiotics 107, 139
Nausea 28, 92, 128
Neurotransmitters 113

O

Oligomeric Proanthocyanidin
(OPC) 64
Olive oil 35
Omega-3 essential fatty
acid 35, 41
Organic food 112
Organic meat 37
Osteoporosis 114, 117
Oxidation 35, 41

P

Parasites 36, 106
PH level 67, 68, 108
Phytonutrients 108
Pine bark extract 64
Plantain 60
Plant sterols 108
Polio cure 65
Popsicles 36
Prayer 113
Pre-digested food 26, 130
Prednisone 16, 17, 20, 26,
44, 114
Pregnancy 19, 69, 132
Primal Defense 108
Probiotics 26, 106, 139
Progesterone cream, natural 45
Prostaglandins 42
Prostate gland 45

Protein 34
    requirements 42
Psychotherapy 113
Purulent skin 61
Pycnogenol 64

Q

Quercetin 66

R

Raw milk 95, 112
Rectal fissures 26, 32, 66
Rectal fistulas
    healing 60
Reishi mushrooms 80
Remission 16, 26, 56
Rice protein 34
Rutin 66

S

Saccharomyces Boulardii 108
Safflower oil 35
Shakes
    mixing 128, 130
Shake recipes
    daily use 86-87
    elemental 40, 70, 83-85
    without Absorb Plus 39
Shunt tube 125, 131
Slippery elm bark 32, 57, 64, 69
Soy protein 34
Spirulina 129
Spiritual healing 113, 135
Splenda 39, 111

Testimonials

After being diagnosed one and a half years ago with indeterminate ulcerative colitis, I tried the full range of conventional 5-ASA drugs (salofalk, asacol, pentasa) but experienced no improvement at all. In fact, some of the drugs worsened my condition. I also tried a number of natural therapies, including restrictive diets such as the Specific Carbohydrate Diet, a wide range of supplements, and bodywork therapies, all of which helped me somewhat, but which I felt did not go far enough toward getting the disease under control.

I decided to try the IBD Remission Diet using Absorb Plus after the onset of a sudden, nasty flare that also resulted in painful swellings on my legs called erythema nodosum that made it difficult for me to walk.

I learned about the IBD Remission Diet after having read Jini Patel Thompson's *Listen To Your Gut*. Although initially I felt skeptical about my ability to stay on a completely liquid diet for any length of time, I decided that it seemed like a much better - and safer - option than the ones my G.I. was offering in the form of steroids and immuno-suppressive drugs.

I followed the diet for two and a half weeks then tapered off the shakes gradually over the course of another one and a half weeks. Within three days of beginning the diet my erythema nodosum began to disappear, and although one does experience some "urgency" as a result of this diet being all liquid - the nearly intolerable urgency I had been experiencing beforehand went away as well. During the course of the diet I never felt hungry, enjoyed the taste of the shakes and was full of energy. I was able to put on and maintain needed weight and was amazed how little self-discipline it took to stay on the diet. I actually found I enjoyed the break from planning menus, shopping, cooking and cleaning up!

Within the first week of returning to solid food I experienced the first solid bowel movements I had had in almost a year. My digestion was quiet and painless and food was properly broken down. My energy levels stayed up and my weight has stayed on.

The IBD Remission Diet has been a dramatic, positive step forward in what I see as an ongoing healing process. Although I may experience flares again in the future, the fear factor is almost gone now that I know I have a powerful tool for managing them that will not cause horrible side effects or damage my immune system. I still consume the shakes on a regular basis, mainly for health and nutritional reasons, but also because I really enjoy them. I would highly recommend this diet for anyone with gastro-intestinal problems or anyone seeking a balanced, natural approach to long-term health.

Emily Donaldson
Toronto, Ontario

Having recently undergone the second of two major surgeries for severe ulcerative colitis, I decided to follow *The IBD Remission Diet* for two weeks with the goal of restoring balance to my gut, losing some weight, and generally "detoxifying" my system.

Absorb Plus is a terrific product and I felt great the whole time I was taking it. The immediate outcome was a reduction in my cravings for caffeine and other stimulants, a huge boost in energy levels, and the loss of an unwanted 12 lbs, which has stayed off. Since my surgeries, I have been prone to painful blockages. After following *The IBD Remission Diet*, my digestion has vastly improved and I have had no blockages at all. This has led me to question whether my surgeries might even have been averted had this elemental diet product and program been available to me earlier.

Craig Small
Toronto, Ontario

LISTEN TO YOUR GUT

Natural healing and dealing with inflammatory bowel disease and irritable bowel syndrome

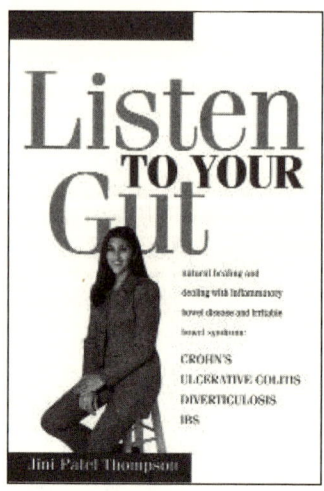

In recent years, more and more people have come to realize that pharmaceutical drugs, surgery, and sophisticated technology cannot provide the keys to health. Many people with Irritable Bowel Syndrome (IBS) and Inflammatory Bowel Diseases like Crohn's, Ulcerative Colitis, and Diverticulitis have already tried the medical treatment protocols, with little success. Until now, very little information has been available on natural, alternative treatments for IBS and IBD. In this revolutionary new book, Jini Patel Thompson presents a series of effective, natural, holistic treatments that work.

She provides detailed and specific information on herbal supplements for quick relief and also long-term healing. She presents a series of Healing Diets designed to relieve and heal the digestive system, step-by-step. Effective lifestyle changes, visualizations, and bodywork therapies are also provided.

With boundless wit and compassion she teaches readers how to control their bowels, transform pain, heal their rectal fissures and relieve gas and bloating. Current popular treatments such as the Gottschall Specific Carbohydrate Diet, Blood Type Diet, Ayurvedic and Chinese Medicine are also discussed

In this inspirational new book, Jini shows readers how to prevent and manage flare-ups using completely natural methods. All levels of symptoms are addressed, from mild gas and diarrhea to intestinal hemorrhaging and severe malnutrition. She explains how the healing process works and guides the reader through the various stages of the journey to health and wholeness.

You can access everything you need to manage and heal your IBD or IBS. This book can show you how.

"I did just one thing suggested in Listen To Your Gut and my diarrhea of ten years stopped within three weeks. I would recommend this book to anyone with these diseases." Catherine Grey

"Conventional medical therapies aren't for everyone, Listen To Your Gut is an excellent tool and resource guide for people looking for viable alternatives." Dr. David Wang BSc, ND, President Finlandia Natural Healing Centre

How does this book differ from *THE IBD REMISSION DIET*, which I already have?

THE IBD REMISSION DIET was written in response to readers of *LISTEN TO YOUR GUT*, who wrote in asking for more detailed instructions on following the Bowel Rest Elemental Diet outlined in Chapter 3 of that book.

LISTEN TO YOUR GUT is a comprehensive compendium of a variety of natural, alternative therapies that work to address specific symptoms of IBD and IBS. *THE IBD REMISSION DIET* however, focuses on just one of those natural therapies (the elemental diet) and then adds a natural supplementation plan to produce an effective program for inducing disease remission.

Whilst *LISTEN TO YOUR GUT* provides you with a variety of treatment options and you put together your own plan based on your individual symptom profile, *THE IBD REMISSION DIET* is a set, step-by-step treatment program that is the same for everyone - the only variable is the length of time you stay on the Diet.

THE IBD REMISSION DIET is the fastest way to heal yourself, but it requires a lot more self-discipline and involves short-term, radical change. You can also attain solid, long-term healing using *LISTEN TO YOUR GUT*, but it usually takes longer to achieve the same results - as you pick and choose from the therapies listed and go at your own pace. Both contain very valuable information and healing tools for healing Crohn's, Ulcerative Colitis, Diverticulitis and Irritable Bowel Syndrome (IBS).

ORDER ONLINE AT: www.caramal.com
ORDER TOLL-FREE: 1-888-866-7745
US$24.95
Hardcover, 256 pgs

RELAX FOR THE FUN OF IT

STRESS RELEASE MADE FUN AND EASY!

A delightful book and CD set to promote humor, relaxation and healing in your life. This cartoon guidebook with voice-guided relaxation exercise will help you release stress and tension from your mind and body. Includes a special relaxation exercise to release tension and emotions from the gut - particularly beneficial for people with IBS and IBD. Open yourself to increased health and joy using this soothing, guided-relaxation CD with accompanying cartoon book. Perfect for yourself or as a gift for loved ones, colleagues and friends.

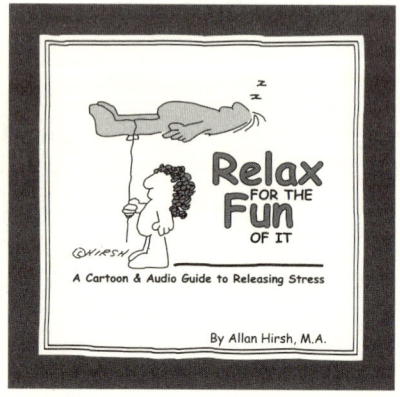

"In my medical and psychotherapy practice, I find that giving patients Allan Hirsh's relaxation exercise can speed their emotional and physical recovery."
Marc Gabel, M.D. Toronto, Ontario

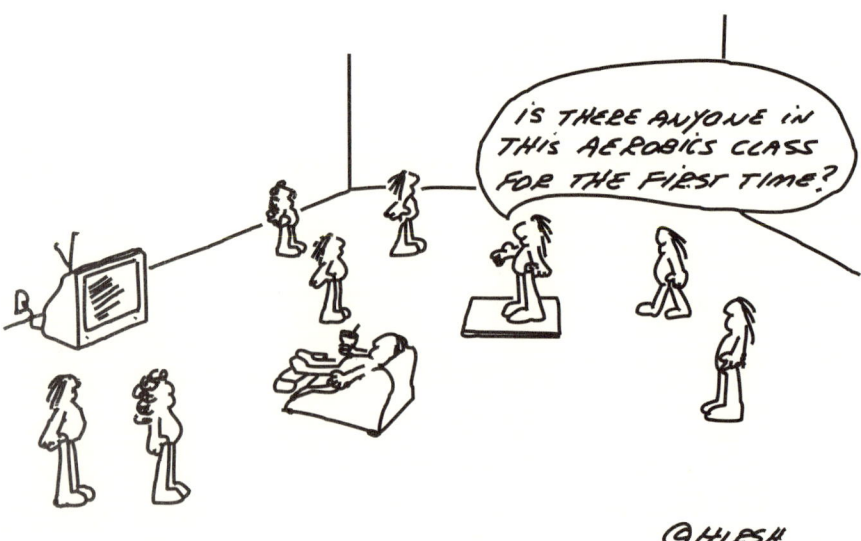

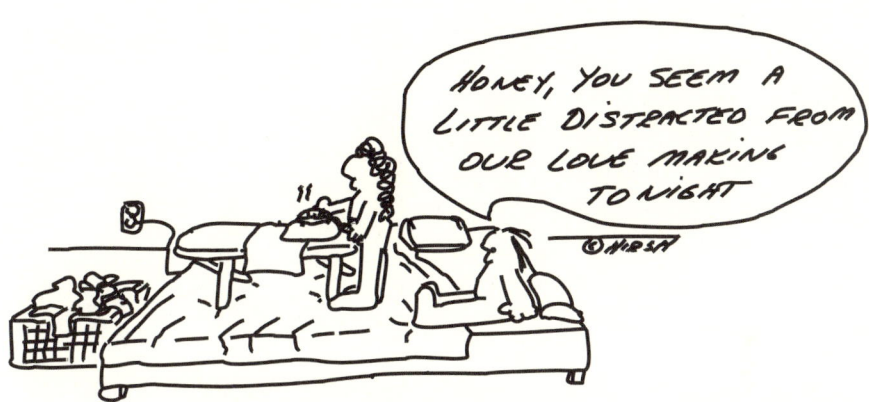

"If we can laugh at our problems, we'll always have something to laugh about. Loving, gentle humor helps us feel lighter and more relaxed. Humor opens the doors that stress, tension and pain have closed. Humor can also help channel stress into something productive. Laughter can provide a distance from pain, which helps us to keep matters in perspective."
Allan Hirsh, M.A.

ORDER ONLINE AT: www.caramal.com
ORDER TOLL-FREE: 1-888-866-7745
US$19.95
Softcover Book and CD
96 pgs. & 2, 16-minute tracks (one with wake-up, one without)

Fill out and mail with your cheque in US$ drawn on a US bank or, a bank draft or, a money order in US dollars made payable to "PSI Fulfillment".

First/Last Name: _____

Mailing Address: _____

City: _____

State/Province: _____

Postal Code: _____

Country: _____

Email Address: _____

Books

LISTEN TO YOUR GUT:
Natural Healing & Dealing with
Inflammatory Bowel Disease &
Irritable Bowel Syndrome
by Jini Patel Thompson _____ x US$24.95 = _____

THE IBD REMISSION DIET:
Achieving Long-Term Health with
An Elemental Diet & Natural
Supplementation Plan
by Jini Patel Thompson _____ x US$24.95 = _____

RELAX FOR THE FUN OF IT:
A Cartoon & Audio Guide to
Releasing Stress
by Allan Hirsh, M.A. _____ x US$19.95 = _____

Choose Shipping:

USPS (USA)	Media Mail	7-10 days	$ 4.00
USPS (Canada)	Int'l Air	5-7 days	$ 7.30
USPS (International)	Global Priority	1-2 weeks	$11.95

Add 8.25% sales tax if you live in Texas to total order,
including shipping and handling: _____

TOTAL COST OF ORDER (books+shipping+tax)
(make cheque out for this amount) _____

Mail your completed form to:
PSI Fulfillment, 8803 Tara Lane, Austin, Texas, 78737 USA

If you have any questions, please call:
1-512-288-5005 or 1-888-866-7745 (Toll-Free USA/Canada only)

Fill out and mail with your cheque in US$ drawn on a US bank or, a bank draft or, a money order in US dollars made payable to "PSI Fulfillment".

First/Last Name: _____

Mailing Address: _____

City: _____

State/Province: _____

Postal Code: _____

Country: _____

Email Address: _____

Books

LISTEN TO YOUR GUT:
Natural Healing & Dealing with
Inflammatory Bowel Disease &
Irritable Bowel Syndrome
by Jini Patel Thompson   _____ x US$24.95 = _____

THE IBD REMISSION DIET:
Achieving Long-Term Health with
An Elemental Diet & Natural
Supplementation Plan
by Jini Patel Thompson   _____ x US$24.95 = _____

RELAX FOR THE FUN OF IT:
A Cartoon & Audio Guide to
Releasing Stress
by Allan Hirsh, M.A.   _____ x US$19.95 = _____

Choose Shipping:

USPS (USA)	Media Mail	7-10 days	$ 4.00
USPS (Canada)	Int'l Air	5-7 days	$ 7.30
USPS (International)	Global Priority	1-2 weeks	$11.95

Add 8.25% sales tax if you live in Texas to total order, including shipping and handling: _____

TOTAL COST OF ORDER (books+shipping+tax)
(make cheque out for this amount)   _____

Mail your completed form to:
PSI Fulfillment, 8803 Tara Lane, Austin, Texas, 78737 USA

If you have any questions, please call:
1-512-288-5005 or 1-888-866-7745 (Toll-Free USA/Canada only)

CARAMAL PUBLISHING

Caramal Publishing Inc.
P.O. Box 29022, Vancouver, B.C., V6J 5C2, Canada
Website: www.caramal.com
Orders: 1-888-866-7745